T0147614

The Great White Hoax

The Suppressed Truth About the
Pharmaceutical Industry
(2nd Edition, Revised)

Robert E. Catalano

iUniverse, Inc.
New York   Bloomington

The Great White Hoax
The Suppressed Truth About the Pharmaceutical Industry

Copyright © 2010 by Robert E. Catalano

All rights reserved. No part of this book may be used or reproduced by any means, graphic, electronic, or mechanical, including photocopying, recording, taping or by any information storage retrieval system without the written permission of the publisher except in the case of brief quotations embodied in critical articles and reviews.

The information, ideas, and suggestions in this book are not intended as a substitute for professional medical advice. Before following any suggestions contained in this book, you should consult your personal physician. Neither the author nor the publisher shall be liable or responsible for any loss or damage allegedly arising as a consequence of your use or application of any information or suggestions in this book.

iUniverse books may be ordered through booksellers or by contacting:

iUniverse
1663 Liberty Drive
Bloomington, IN 47403
www.iuniverse.com
1-800-Authors (1-800-288-4677)

Because of the dynamic nature of the Internet, any Web addresses or links contained in this book may have changed since publication and may no longer be valid. The views expressed in this work are solely those of the author and do not necessarily reflect the views of the publisher, and the publisher hereby disclaims any responsibility for them.

ISBN: 978-1-4502-2128-3 (sc)
ISBN: 978-1-4502-2129-0 (ebook)

Printed in the United States of America

iUniverse rev. date: 06/23/2010

Table of Contents

1. Introduction

In the United States, a trillion dollars a year is spent on a burgeoning medical industry that proudly proclaims again and again, using the most sophisticated media techniques, its medical miracles. Yet, the real truth is conveniently left behind. Hundreds of thousands of drugs now pollute the bloodstream of the nation. We see some people living to well over 100 years of age, but the average lifespan for those medically oriented is much less. The economy of the nation has been destroyed and part of that destruction is due to high medical costs. In an effort to purchase health and longevity we have bought for ourselves sin, disease, crime, sickness, death and financial ruin. If the medical industry had not been caught up in the profit-frenzy of drugs and medicine, we would have virtually no disease today, and for what little we might have, we would have a cure.

The author of this book does not claim any training or expertise in any aspect of American medicine or any other medicine. Everything herein, unless otherwise noted, is his personal opinion, study and observation, with information gathered from various sources for more than half a century. Unlike the medical industry, he has no agenda. He has no statistics. He has performed no laboratory studies. He does not sell herbs. He does not sell grains. He does not sell vitamins or magic potions. He does not endorse any product that is sold to cure or help cure or to prevent or help prevent any disease or disorder. He has nothing to sell but this book and he recognizes the possibility that he may not for long be allowed to make his opinions public.

Basic health cannot be bought. It is a gift from the great Creator. Along with that gift, comes the body's innate ability to prevent disease and to keep itself healthy. No drugs, chemicals, antibiotics, vaccines or other morbid matter, when introduced into the human bloodstream can improve on the vast powers of that amazing gift.

It is a known fact that the human body has the ability to heal itself. It has been known to prevent and deal successfully with just about every disease known to the human race. All it requires is reasonable care, good nutrition, and sufficient air and water. There is often nothing to buy. We should usually avoid those who have something to sell. The basic need of the human body is to be nourished and free from toxins. Of course, psychological, physical and social circumstances should be taken into account. A good holistic practitioner who sees the person as a whole, can be beneficial. In today's society, organic stuff, water filters, alkaline minerals and natural supplements can also be part of the solution; but nothing is more important than to protect the body from trauma and to keep it free from the intake of toxins, poisons, recreational drugs, artificial substances, and most importantly, medicinal drugs and vaccines.

What the medical experts refer to as the immune system is actually the human body itself. It houses one of the greatest forces known to man. This force whose main component is the bloodstream, which flows through thousands of miles of arteries every minute, has been known to cure any and every disease from the common cold to the worst cancer. In spite of this fact, the medical authorities concentrate on their search for drugs. The search for the magic bullet that never was and never will be is a very profitable business. Charlatans across the earth and through the ages have taken advantage of the great human frailty of self-indulgence. The desire of the people for a quick fix, a magic bullet, some kind of procedure, a packaged product or maybe even a prayer to some obscure deity is often preferable to the surrender of a self-indulgent lifestyle. The bloodstream is a dynamic entity. It does its finest work in a pristine condition. The most dreaded cancers, diseases and infections have been cured by the workings of a highly tuned immune system, an entity that is self-cleansing, self-healing and self-sufficient while requiring only air, water, and nutrition.

It is outrageous to believe that the introduction of filth into the human bloodstream is beneficial either in the prevention of disease or to the healing process. Any morbid matter introduced into the bloodstream damages the immune system, sometimes to the extent of limiting the body's ability to prevent disease or to heal itself. I find, with no exception to the rule, that any drug or vaccination used either in the treatment or prevention of disease is a total fraud.

Every packaged product other than normal nutrition is usually a means of separating the non-thinking brainwashed person from his or her money and often his or her health, while at the same time causing a hoard of problems for society at large. The magic bullet to prevent disease or enhance health goes back to the beginning of time. It is also the foundation of our multi-billion dollar pharmaceutical industry —an industry that is destroying the American economy as well as the American bloodstream. It is the self-indulgence of man that makes him search for a non-existent product or procedure to solve his physical or even his mental and emotional problems.

The medical industry has taken full advantage of this human frailty. They not only create and supply a multitude of products and procedures; they have learned to use highly sophisticated means of brainwashing, to brainwash the public and insure for themselves a giant share of the American pocketbook.

I have found from my own study and observations that most accepted medical treatments that include operations, testing, and other highly promoted procedures, are unnecessary, harmful, and sometimes fatal.

I will not discuss the surgical part of the industry that does have some iota of redeeming grace. However, I will concentrate on the pharmaceutical industry, which I have found to be almost completely useless, outrageous and bordering on the criminal. Penicillin, Achromycin (tetracycline), nearly all the great wonder drugs, antibiotics and nearly every other medicinal drug that is purported to cure or prevent our illnesses, do nothing but maim and kill, and at the very best, subdue the immune system so as to slow down the body's natural power of healing and immunity.

The only reason for the veil of secrecy that surrounds the medical industry is to hide the scam that takes place within. I dedicate this book to exposing the outrage being perpetrated on the American people and the people of the world by the drug industry. The belief that poison can be beneficial to one's health is one of the greatest examples of brainwashing of our time, possibly of all time.

Health comes from the body's innate ability to protect and heal itself. The drug sellers entice our elected officials into a cozy relationship. Then by brainwashing the public through excessive, meaningless advertising and self-serving statistics, they merely take credit for the good results that come from natural healing, which often comes in spite of their "treatment" while at the same time, creating for themselves an image of respectability. All that is necessary for the medical industry to succeed is "treatment". "Treatment" which rarely works! "Treatment" that rarely ever did work and seldom will!

The US Government, in league with the medical industry continues to approve, endorse and promote drugs. Where do they get this knowledge of medicine and pharmaceutical products? I venture to say they obtain it from the drug lobbyists more than anyone else. The drug industry has more representatives in Congress than the American people have representing them! Outrageous, obscene and insulting! Since 1998, drug companies have spent $758 million on lobbying —more than any other industry, according to government records analyzed by the Center for Public Integrity, a watchdog group. In Washington, the industry has 1,274 lobbyists —more than two for every member of Congress.

Hundreds of thousands of drugs now pollute the bloodstream of the nation. Every medicine chest in America is chock-full of drugs, all in the name of health. Senior citizens are hit the hardest. Seniors not only suffer the diseases created by these products; they are ruined financially by the cost. The elderly in America are feeble, ill, and decrepit. The elderly are plagued with Parkinson's disease, Alzheimer's; the list goes on. The elderly in America suffer poor health, not because they are old, but because they are drugged and may have through life-long ignorance, made bad food and beverage choices. The doctor's job should be to enhance the immune system —not to pollute it. The fact that every Senior Citizen in America takes as many as 20 medicines a day is a feather in the cap of the pharmaceutical sales force; but the drugging of the elderly in America is a national catastrophe.

Approving more drugs for cancer borders on the criminal. Not only are medicinal drugs the cause of most cancer, they are also the reason that cancer is not curable. Cures are taking place at this time, but mainly by those who dare to buck the system. The medical authorities still remain disinterested in any 'cure' which cannot be marketed, or does not have to be dispensed in a medical facility. For that reason, cancer research has gone 100 years without a cure! The longstanding claim that the cure is on the horizon has proven to be either a falsehood or a mirage.

Most of the populace has been brainwashed into believing that pharmaceutical products can cure or prevent disease. The present goal of the pharmaceutical industry is to bring every American into the fold, by force, if necessary. Americans may soon be drugged, electro-shocked, vaccinated and operated on by government mandate or court order with police or military enforcement. Forced medicine is not an easy accomplishment in a free society; but headway is being made in that direction. The medical gurus are getting their way. In spite of parental rebellion, children are now forced to get vaccinated. Parents who withhold chemotherapy from their children stand to be prosecuted. Chemotherapy treatment, one of the vilest, most useless, most immune-damaging, cancer-causing and cancer-enhancing concoctions is now becoming the law of the land. This is the power of brainwashing and political contributions and of a Congress that has dedicated itself to serving big business. When death follows the refusal of a parent for their child's chemotherapy, the police can now be brought into the picture. When someone dies a horrible death after chemotherapy treatment under medical supervision, which is an everyday occurrence, the medical industry has automatic and total exoneration.

I have found that chemotherapy and/or radiation interferes with the remission of cancer by weakening the immune system. It is a fact, admitted by the medical authorities, that the best defense against cancer is a healthy immune system; yet, today's chemotherapy treatment weakens the immune system, often to the point of no return, causing the cancer to become a disease of the entire bloodstream. Thus by administering these vile products to a cancer patient, the doctor could be guilty of legalized murder. This presents no problem for the doctor. He is completely exonerated without investigation of any kind. Should a Christian Scientist use prayer as preferred treatment, it had better appear to succeed, or indictment and prosecution will be swift. This is the power of the medical industry, its deep pockets, and a Congress that because of greed and ignorance, has turned its back on the American people.

How did the medical industry get this far? First and most importantly, by political contributions. Millions of dollars are given to our Congressmen by the medical industry every year. The pharmaceutical lobby has more lobbyists than there are members of Congress. It had a combined lobbying and campaign contribution budget in 1999 and 2000 of $197 million dollars! Larger than any other industry. Secondly, many of the same congressmen who accept donations from the drug industry, also invest in drug company stocks. Any vote that favors the drug company also favors the stock portfolio of the congressman. For that reason, our representatives are taken up with protecting, promoting and accommodating the drug industry. It gets them in office, and makes them rich once they get there! Since 1998 drug companies have spent hundreds of millions of dollars on lobbying and hundreds of millions on extensive television advertising promotions the likes of which are generally unknown in other countries.

Next to politicians promoting the medical industry, self-serving statistics are the great pillar of the medical fiasco. When someone dies because of a medication, which is more common than is believable, it is rarely attributed to the medication. Doctors are well versed in what to do. For instance, when a person dies from the flu shot, which is an every day occurrence, the death certificate might easily read — "heart failure."

The drug corporations can easily afford to lobby thousands of state legislators and federal and state bureaucrats to pass laws that will force us to buy their products, and that is exactly what the industry is planning for us at this time. It is the mandatory feature of these products that will make them so profitable in the future. Former President Bush, and much of the Congress, in league with the drug industry, passed onto their successors pending legislation that will force the American People to accept medical treatment by government mandate.

The drug companies are not only guilty of a great physical assault on the American people; they have become the worst enemy of the nation's economy. A trillion-dollar a year health care bill has made America weak. A rich nation now finds itself poor. A great people are brought to their knees and made to grovel. Not by a foreign power, but by an enemy within!

There is a place for the medical industry in our society. Although I have found there are thousands of unnecessary operations and other medical procedures taking place in hospitals every day all over this country, I have also seen miracles performed on the operating table. Especially in man-made disorders, where certain physical assistance was necessary before the body's built-in power could take over its business of healing. However the rushing of a patient to the operating table with a disease or disorder that can be successfully dealt with by the body's own natural built-in mechanism is nothing but self-serving and outrageous, and possibly more sinister than that. I can also say, firmly and without any question in my mind, that there is very little place in the world society for the pharmaceutical industry. In spite of giant strides made in some areas of health care such as emergency services, hernia repair, birth tumors, organ, limb and body part repair and replacement and burn therapy among others, the drug industry will prove to be the Number One enemy of the world. We must stop this villain in its acquisition of power!

We must stop the drug industry from drafting government policy. We must stop political contributions and other forms of payment to our government officials by the drug companies. We must rise from out of our stupor and realize that 100 years of cancer research without a cure is not an excellent record. Cancer research is a great failure, and should be treated as such. When we awake from the mind control of the medical industry we see that the billions of dollars being poured into organizations such as the American Cancer Society do not go for research but simply to fatten up the bankrolls of the Society's executive officers and their cronies. This is an outrage and a sham and could only be tolerated by a brainwashed populace and the elected officials and media who have sold them out.

The United States is Number One in the use of medicinal drugs and spends $2 trillion annually for a system with the highest infant mortality and lowest after-sixty life expectancy among industrialized nations. More proof that medicine is the cause, not the cure. It is estimated that in America in 2007, nearly $2 trillion was spent on health care. Despite this massive expenditure on treatment, more Americans are sicker than ever before with diseases that are largely preventable. Why is the amount of money being spent on prevention just a pittance compared with the amount spent on treatment? The answer is simple —when you are sick it is highly profitable to various giant corporations. When you are well, it does not profit them much at all.

I have found medical research to be a farce. Government researchers accept thousands of dollars from the drug companies. University Professors doing medical studies are also on the receiving end of drug company benefits. Payments from the drug companies go to every rung of the educational, political and corporate ladder. No stone is left unturned.

Medical statistics are the reason for the success of vaccinations, antibiotics, and all other medicines. Whether these drugs work or not is determined by medical statistics. Where do these statistics come from? Entirely from the people who are in the business of promoting these products; and because of the power of the medical lobby, medical statistics have become the law of the land. Because of the power of brainwashing by excessive advertising, the power of political contributions, and the power of the freedom to create self-serving statistics, Americans are led to believe, and sometimes even forced to believe, that the thousands of poisons, being promoted by the drug industry and soon to be forced on them by law, are beneficial to their health.

2. Statistics

I have no interest in statistics produced by those who have an agenda. Statistics can be made to say whatever they are wanted to say. Unless statistics are well documented and the documentation concise and researched by those who have no vested interest in the outcome of the study, they might just as well be outright lies, which they usually are. According to Mark Twain: *"There are three kinds of lies: lies, damned lies, and "statistics."* Lies are not allowed in most spheres. Damned lies are probably worse somehow and still not allowed. Statistics however, were made to order for the medical industry.

With the magic of numbers they can lie without getting into trouble! I do not provide the public with statistics that have resulted from my own findings. It would be an insult since statistics can be made to achieve any desired result. The drug industry with their cronies at the CDC and FDA know this all too well. The FDA could use a 5-person study to test a drug; and if 2 persons survived, it could be considered a 40% success; but the cries of thousands of people who have no question that their children acquired autism from vaccination are considered invalid and not sufficient for a finding.

The medical authorities can usually achieve their desired results; but in any case they are prepared to readily provide statistics for any question that might come their way. They have ever-present statistics for why a drug might work or why a vaccine is necessary; but they can never produce proof that their products or services are beneficial. If a patient survives, "He responded to treatment" If he succumbs, "He died from complications." They have ready-made answers.

The unwritten rule and apparently the first one learned in medical school is that the patient never dies from treatment whether it be surgeries, drugs or whatever else. The fact is the patient almost always dies from the treatment. Poison is not very beneficial to the human constitution! The patient dies from "complications," says the doctor. "Complications", another trick medical word with little or no meaning. When doctors are called on to produce documented statistics or findings, there is a large silence. If a study is actually done and the results are not satisfactory, any reason can be used to reject the study; and they may keep rejecting studies until the results are satisfactory. So why bother studying? They don't bother! Not very much! So interwoven is the drug industry with the media and our elected officials that it has become untouchable.

The pharmaceutical industry with their friends at the CDC and FDA deals greatly in statistics. Cure is not necessary. Successful treatment is not required, all that is required are the medical statistics taken from thin air and readily accepted by a brainwashed public. Statistics are the backbone and foundation of the medical industry. Statistics provided by the FDA prove "beyond the shadow of a doubt" that poison can be beneficial to one's health! If medical statistics were compiled by statisticians who had no interest in the outcome, the drug industry would topple into the dust.

No doctor ever declined to quote statistics. How often does a doctor say, "Excuse me while I check the statistics?" Never! No doctor ever has had to research statistics. Statistics are ever present and have lain on the tip of the doctor's tongue since the beginning of time. I have come to the conclusion that doctors use statistics strictly for support, not for illumination.

Most of the Western World's population is self-indulgent. They welcome the quick fix that will deal with their ailments. They not only welcome it, they demand it. The pharmaceutical industry is only too happy to oblige. They do research to the tune of billions of dollars, not looking for a cure, but looking for anything that would be toxic enough to require control by the authorities. Requiring a prescription means more income for the industry. A non-toxic substance would still be profitable; but not profitable enough, so as to satisfy the appetite of a ravenous industry. A medicine or poison must be slow acting enough so it will be accepted as beneficial by a brainwashed or confused public. Although slow-acting poisons are approved by the FDA, it retains the appearance of respectability by disapproving fast-acting poisons. Cure is not required by the drug companies nor is cure necessary for approval by the FDA.

The medical industry has become so powerful that cure is not even necessary to receive payment for services. The word "cure" is no longer part of the medical vocabulary. All that is required of a product is that it be toxic enough so that it will require a doctor's prescription. Far removed from its original purpose, the FDA's job is to approve poison for human consumption and to distinguish slow acting poisons from fast acting poisons.

Beware of medical advertising. It is responsible for a large part of the industry's budget. Meaningless excessive medical advertising, that includes words or phrases with little or no meaning, confuse the listener and gives the appearance of respectability. Use of such vague terms as "treatment", "giant strides", "check with your doctor", and "complications" have been found by the drug promoters to be an excellent method of brainwashing while achieving for them the appearance of respectability. Much of the advertising during the News Hours is paid for by drug companies. Much of the newscast is focused on the wonders of medicine. Every day a new wonder drug is presented that may be the key to salvation, but of course, it never is.

The drug companies, having brought the FDA and CDC into the fold, as well as our elected officials, have now become a law unto themselves and the law of the land. These agencies that were formed to serve the American people, now give their allegiance to the medical industry. The medical industry is preparing itself to draft government policy. It is not so bad for those who have been brainwashed into believing that drugs are the key to health and longevity; but for those of us still caught in the act of thinking, there is the feeling of terror that these vile products may be forced on us, our children or even our household pets by an industry running rampant with power.

Statistics are gathered by the medical industry, not to get to the truth, but to promote an agenda. Statistics can be made to show whatever is desired. If a group of researchers is studying a certain drug, unsatisfactory results can be discarded for any reason. There is no reason to keep unsatisfactory results, not unless, of course, they were seeking the truth. Testing may be repeated until the desired results are achieved. Thousands of parents cry out in horror as their children are maimed and killed by vaccinations. I have, myself, received dozens of letters from such parents. They are immediately rebuffed by the authorities that accept only whatever facts, figures and statistics are acceptable to their own agenda. The outcry of thousands of parents who swear that their children acquired autism from vaccination is not good enough for the medical authorities to admit a possible link between the vaccine and the disease. I suggest that as the numbers of such claims grow, and they will continue to grow, the cries of these parents will still fall on deaf ears.

Once again, I ignore statistics compiled by those who have an agenda. But I can say that from my own observations, I find that vaccinations and drugs are not only worthless; they are harmful and often fatal. Vaccinations positively are the cause of autism, tumors, epilepsy, asthma, Alzheimer's and other diseases too numerous to mention.

The medical industry guarantees nothing. What they do is maintain that cure is possible with or without their intervention; but of course, medical statistics say, "chances are better with medicinal drugs and medical services than without". If and when a person under medical treatment happens to recover from his or her aliment, the drugs and medical procedures that were administered to the patient receive the credit. These experts often have the audacity to quote exact statistics and percentages to show the value of their products or services. To question medical statistics can be considered un-American. In a court of law it could amount to contempt.

The immune system, a mind-boggling multi-faceted force which includes a mechanism that protects and defends the body against disease is not only a self-healing entity, it has been know to cure every disease under the sun. This fact alone could decapitate the drug industry. All cures are performed by the immune system. From the beginning of time, charlatans have duped the ignorant, into believing that some substance or some procedure was necessary to prevent sickness or achieve a cure. These were the first doctors. They would usually introduce some concoction to the patient. If the patient stayed well or healed, the doctor would take credit for what was actually the body's natural power of immunity or built-in healing ability. There were concoctions used to ward off disease. These were akin to the first vaccinations.

Diseases can be prevented and cured only by the immune system. The search for a magic bullet goes on to this day by a brainwashed people who are taken advantage of by an industry that has been given unlimited power. Diseases the doctors cannot claim to cure (practically all diseases) are now "treated". No proof is necessary to determine whether the treatment is or is not beneficial. All that is necessary are once again, "medical statistics." This patient died in one month after treatment. "But" says the doctor, "He would have died in two weeks without the treatment", and once again the notation reads, "Responded to treatment." "Treatment has prolonged this patient's life" according to the doctor and his "statistics". "Treatment has helped to cure this aliment". If the doctor says so, it must be true! When the person expires after his so called treatment, "He lived as long as he did because of the treatment". When a patient dies a horrible death after his chemotherapy, "It would have been more horrible without treatment", so say the doctors with their ever present "statistics". Where is the basis for all these statistics? I have searched high and low to no avail. There are no worthwhile statistics anywhere on this planet to prove that drugs are of any value in the treatment or prevention of disease. The only proof of value is found in the "studies" and "statistics" of the drug promoters. Many people, of course, will claim that drugs benefit them. Example: Prescription drugs or even over the counter medicine often masks symptoms and hence, these drugs appear to 'cure' or provide relief.

When I inquired as to how many children with curable diseases, die in hospitals each year while under medical treatment, I was told that this was not important enough for them to keep records. The medical people aren't counting. They had no reason to know. I found later, that someone was counting. The fact is that the number of children who die in hospitals each year with curable diseases is astronomical.

How many people survive with cancer, even advanced cancer, and yet refused medical intervention? The medical authorities say "Very few." Where do they get this information? As usual, from thin air. There are no such records. The authorities don't know. It is of no concern to them. Their business is selling drugs and operations. The largest part of their business is testing. Testing for diseases for which they have no cure! The fact is that the real cures of the worst diseases, several of which I have personally witnessed and participated in, (below see "Letters", Idaho Observer November 15, 2005) are usually by those who reject medical treatment; and especially by those who reject medicinal drugs. I have also found that the longest living AIDS patients were those who refused drug therapy. Anything that has the ability to self-heal should be allowed and encouraged to self-heal; and that means just about everything. Whether it is the common cold or cancer, Nature does the work. The doctor does very little of any benefit; but Nature is seldom given the credit.

I am not sure AIDS is reversible. It is very similar to cancer and may be a condition where the immune system is too far damaged to achieve remission. If AIDS can be reversed, I am certain the reversal is similar for cancer. A stringent alkaline regimen that forms a condition within the body where cancer cells cannot thrive.

The two magical words that keep the pharmaceutical industry in business are "treatment" and "statistics". These are the words that cost US citizens more than a trillion dollars a year plus ill health, pain, suffering, crime and even environmental pollution.

Are statistics provided by Harvard and other such institutions independent of the medical industry? I doubt it. The drug industry in 1991 alone, gave over $2 billion to colleges and universities for research. The drug industry is not a slouch. They hover over us like exactly what they are: the monster that we have created and allow to exist. Medical schools have long been corrupted by Big Pharma, which secretly bribes professors with meals, gifts, vacations and cash bonuses to make sure they teach students a pro-pharmaceutical curriculum.

Now some medical students are fed up with the corruption, and they are demanding that schools require professors to disclose their financial ties with drug companies. Unbelievably, the medical schools are refusing!

Harvard Medical Students Rebel Against Big Pharma Ties

By Pollywog

"Two hundred Harvard Medical School students are confronting the school's administration, demanding an end to pharmaceutical industry influence in the classroom.

"The students worry that pharmaceutical industry scandals in recent years, including criminal convictions, billions of dollars in fines, proof of bias in research and publishing and false marketing claims, have cast a bad light on the medical profession. The students have criticized Harvard as being less vigilant than other leading medical schools in monitoring potential financial conflicts by faculty members.

"Harvard received the lowest possible grade, an "F," from the American Medical Student Association, a national group that rates how well medical schools monitor and control drug industry money.

"The students were joined by Dr. Marcia Angell, a faculty member and former editor-in-chief of the New England Journal of Medicine, who has vigorously advocated for an end to liaisons between academia and Big Pharma."

Source: Alliance for Human Research Protection. March 3, 2009

3. Drugs

A drug rarely is of any value in the cure of disease. It may sometimes have value in the suppression or relief, but almost never in the cure. Every drug is harmful. Prescription for medicine is a prescription for poison. Penicillin, antibiotics, sulfa drugs, and the other thousands of drugs, including the "life-saving" drugs that sit on drug store shelves and are found in every medicine chest of every American household, are completely worthless and all are harmful. Drugs that artificially control blood pressure, fever, heartbeat and other bodily functions, simply interfere with the natural workings of the body. The human body has a built-in brain mechanism that knows exactly how to deal with any innate physical problem. It can send into remission any disease or disorder, from the common cold to the worst cancer. Prevention or Cure never comes because of drugs and it does not come in a packaged product. Good results may come in spite of drugs and other concoctions, but never because of them. The intake of poison can in no way contribute to good health. When the human body fails to deal successfully with a disease or disorder, no doctor with pills or needle in hand, can improve on the workings of the amazing bloodstream.

Nearly all disease germs are found within the human body. They become activated when suppression or damaging of the immune system occurs, which is exactly what happens when we take medicine. The human body acts positively to normal amounts of air, water and good nutrition; and negatively to the intake of most other substances. Acidic food and products in reasonable amounts are acceptable and even necessary to the human body; but an imbalanced diet high in acidic foods such as animal protein, sugar, caffeine, and processed foods tends to disrupt the body's balance making people prone to chronic and degenerative disease. The cure for cancer, arthritis and practically everything else, is first to eliminate the cause, which in our society, is often overuse of coffee, alcohol, and other acidic foods and unnatural products. Frequently, medicinal drugs cause disease. It is usually not difficult to find the cause of an ailment, but in some cases the cause is not obvious. It may sometimes be necessary to search.

The next step is to create an alkaline environment within the body where disease cannot flourish. This is best done by means of a highly alkaline or vegetarian diet. Fruits and vegetables are alkaline. More importantly one should usually avoid highly acidic foods, chemicals, and especially medicinal drugs. We find that disease is more prevalent in the older population because the older a person becomes, the more his or her immune system has been weakened by medicine.

Medicine is often prescribed for a person on the first trip to the doctor, and that person usually continues taking medicine until the end of life. There are also other toxins in our society that are damaging to the human body, but medicine is the great crippler. More than 100 years ago Dr. Henry Lindlahr put it best: *"... the poisons and serums employed to arrest the disease process very often affect vital parts and organs permanently, causing the gradual deterioration of cells and tissues, and paving the way for tuberculosis, chronic affection of the kidneys, cancer, etc., in later years."*

Before the great rush to medicine, tuberculosis or cancer and other diseases were usually caused by overloading the system with meat, coffee, alcohol or tobacco; but as soon as these bad habits were discontinued, and the organs of elimination were stimulated by natural methods, the encumbrances were eliminated, and the much-dreaded symptoms subsided and disappeared, often with surprising rapidity.

The populace, today, is so brainwashed that even those who have learned to avoid the vile poisons known as medicinal drugs, still ask, "What can I take for this ailment?" They continue to be duped, not only by the doctors, but also by some holistic practitioners who have products to sell.

Alternate therapies are often no better than mainstream medicine. There are many on TV, radio and in the media who will sell us our health. The fact is they have little to sell and there is little that we should buy. Health comes from within. Like all bodily diseases, whether it is a plain simple skin rash or a cancerous tumor, it can be cured by the body's natural built-in healing ability. All diseases have been known to vanish as mysteriously as they appeared.

The medical authorities, when cornered, will admit this fact; but they have no interest in solving the mystery of diseases that vanish for no apparent reason. They have no interest in a cure that does not involve medical products or procedures. For that reason they have found no cure for anything. Not for the common cold, not for cancer and not for anything in between. A cure can never be found in a chemical laboratory or on a drug store shelf. As for polio, the one and only disease where the medical industry claims total victory, the boast is a complete farce. Not true. Study has shown that the polio vaccine was the cause of the problem. Not the solution. The medical authorities have only one interest. That is in promoting their agenda. The medical industry, in spite of the Hippocratic Oath and all other embellishments, is exactly what its name implies, an *"Industry!"*

The vilest substances known to man are touted by the drug companies and approved by the US government through the FDA, whose job, unbelievable as it sounds, is mainly to approve poison for human consumption. However, do not take my word for it. The absolute proof is in the PDR —the "Physicians Desk Reference", either in printed form or electronically on-line. The evils of all patent drugs are clearly delineated in this massive "biblical" epic produced by Merck for the drug industry. The PDR is the verbatim statements provided by all drug manufacturers describing the use and warnings associated with all their concoctions. Adverse reaction warnings that range from an innocuous headache to suicidal tendencies to death. Indeed, medicine is far worse than the malady. Equally shocking is the fact that the finely printed inserts that accompany over the counter drugs often do not reveal all the shocking truths. Only the PDR tells all —usually. Drugs are approved that kill, maim, pollute and are capable of causing just about every disease known to man. The important business of the FDA is to approve drugs that can be peddled by the drug industry. These products are nothing less than slow-acting poison for human consumption.

In approving drugs, the FDA does not consider cure to be a prerequisite. If cure were a prerequisite no drug could ever get approved. All that is necessary for approval by the FDA is that the disease that can be caused by these products is slow enough so as not to be apparent. When we place a pill into our mouth, it is not usually enough for a quick death; but it is positively the beginning of a disease and a slow death. Americans are taking pills and Americans are being slowly poisoned.

The agenda of the medical industry is to slowly poison, operate on, electroshock or "treat", not cure, but treat, in one way or another, every person on the planet; and, when necessary, to accomplish this feat by government mandate and by force. All this in the name of profits and power.

The process of spontaneous remission and natural immunity is one that exists. It is the built-in mechanism used by the body to protect and heal itself. So powerful is the medical industry that a person must fight, sometimes in the courts, for the right to employ natural healing in preference to medicinal drugs or operations or other medical procedures. If the doctor is asked,

"Can a patient be immunized or recover without the use of medicine?" The answer is well rehearsed, "Yes, health can be acquired without the use of medicinal products and procedures; but statistics favor medical procedures." "Statistics" that come from thin air are the backbone and foundation of the medical industry. Statistics, taken from thin air have now become the law of the land, thanks to our "statesmen" who occupy the halls of Congress.

There is no medicinal drug in the world and seldom a packaged product that has ever been of value in the healing process. No vaccine, drug, antibiotic or other pharmaceutical product has ever failed to produce its share of horror. Once again, the medical industry creates and keeps only the records that promote its agenda. Honest statistics are not to be found. True and honest statistics would destroy the medical industry as we know it today.

The intake of any and every drug whether legal or illegal, is the first step in producing disease. The next drug, and there is always a next drug, would be the second step. The more medicine we take, the closer we move to disease and death. The only things that appear to be more harmful than illegal drugs are the legal ones. I have found that the number one cause of disease in our society today, including cancer, is medicinal drugs. I have also found that illicit drugs don't come close to causing the number of deaths caused by prescription drugs. The human body rebels at the thought of medicine. It does not want it. It does not want it to interfere with its own built-in mechanism for healing and prevention of disease. The first pill a person takes is the first step towards disease or what the doctor politely refers to as a "side effect". Of course the second pill is the second step toward a side effect, and so on, until the patient has enough side effects so as to be labeled "disease". Medicine actually produces disease. The doctor's business, of course, now escalates. The first disease now requires treatment. Not cure, but treatment, which means possibly a medical procedure, but very often, another drug.

The word "cure" has been long forgotten by an industry running rampant. Cure is not important. It is not considered. It is sometimes not even possible because of a medicine-damaged bloodstream. Because of a brainwashed public, cure is completely unnecessary for the industry to gather in their usual enormous profits. When healing does occur in spite of drug poisoning, the doctor chalks that one up as a victory for medicine. Actually it is a victory for the immune system. The immune system is sometimes so powerful that in can defeat both the disease and the medical chemical assault. The medical industry has perfected, not the science of healing, but the science of drug promotion and profits. Complete healing, especially noticeable in the elderly, never arrives. The physical problems of the elderly continue to escalate because of their great intake of "medicine". Each drug is the beginning of a new disease that requires more treatment that often means another drug. The elderly never enjoy a clean bill of health. As they take more and more drugs, they suffer more and more ailments until they die of, according to the authorities, "Old Age!"

So laden are the elderly with medicinal drugs that at the time of death, it is not uncommon to find as many as twenty different medicines at their bedside, with death caused by as many different diseases. The body's natural healing process is a great accommodation to the drug industry; but it seldom receives any recognition. The stage has been set. The script has been written. Credit for any healing or remission which might occur in spite of the poisons being administered by the health professionals, is chalked up to the drugs. Drugs get the credit, and a brainwashed public agrees that drugs seem to have been successful.

The real drug pushers sit in fancy offices of many of the great drug companies and send fat checks out to their agents dressed in clean white coats prescribing hundreds of mind and immune-altering drugs. These include narcotics, sedatives, tranquilizers and hundreds of other destructive, and often habit-forming, drugs. Drug companies are known to pay doctors thousands of dollars, simply to prescribe their particular products. Many doctors often comply, knowing that what they prescribe cures nothing and is nothing other than slow poisoning. Since one drug is just as good as another, or should I say "just as bad", it is not unusual for the doctor to cooperate with the drug manufacturer, prescribe the drug manufacturer's particular product, and receive a big fat check. Patients clamoring for a drug "fix" further exacerbate this egregious situation. Even when doctors prefer not recommending a drug, they also know that if they do not provide the prescription, they will lose business —patients will simply go to another drug pusher because it is easier to take a pill than take responsibility for life style changes that could prevent illness in the first place. This is how brainwashed unthinking people have become.

As Doctors Write Prescription, Drug Company Writes a Check

By Gardiner Harris, New York Times, June 27, 2004

(excerpt)

"The check for $10,000 arrived in the mail unsolicited. The doctor who received it from the drug maker Schering-Plough said it was made out to him personally in exchange for an attached "consulting" agreement that required nothing other than his commitment to prescribe the company's medicines. Two other physicians said in separate interviews that they, too, received checks unbidden from Schering-Plough, one of the world's biggest drug companies".

If this were an isolated incident, it would be just that, an isolated incident; but *"According to the U.S. General Accountability Office, drug companies spent $16 billion on direct marketing to physicians in the United States in 2001, more than $19,000 per physician."* (Melissa M. Stiles, MD; Bruce Barrett, MD, PHD; American Family Physician, May 15, 2007).

I have heard that some doctors have received as much as $100,000 or more. It sounds unbelievable to me, too. I stand ready to be corrected; but no one is stepping forward to do the correcting.

"In 1998 Big Pharma went to the US Food & Drug Administration (FDA) and got permission to advertise drugs, drugs, and more drugs directly to the American consumer. Their intent appeared to be: (1) sell more drugs to the American consumer, and, (2) control the media, especially US television." —Tim Bolen, Bolen Report. The real intent appears brainwashing of the American People through excessive and meaningless advertising! Meaningless and excessive drug advertising is also designed to create an image of respectability for the pharmaceutical industry. Just a reminder, and thanks to our elected officials, drug ads

are illegal in nearly every country in the world except, of course, the US.

How important is it for the drug companies to promote their products? Why is brainwashing so important to the drug manufacturers? Drugs promoted by the manufacturer and pushed by the doctors can produce billions of dollars. Annual sales of some of the top best-selling drugs that cure nothing but have the ability to cause a multitude of the worst diseases known to man:

Lipitor — $12 billion

Plavix — $6 billion

Nexium — $6 billion

Advair — $5 billion

Zocor — $5 billion

Despite the bad publicity regarding Merck's deadly Vioxx painkiller, which allegedly has killed more Americans than the entire Vietnam War, Gardasil, Zostavax, and Rotateq were all vaccines introduced by Merck in an attempt to turn their finances around in the wake of litigation over thousands of deaths allegedly caused by the painkiller Vioxx.

The FDA has approved Merck's Gardasil vaccine, which allegedly prevents cervical cancer, by adding it to a list of recommended shots for girls ages 11 and 12. This is more proof that these agencies are serving the drug industry rather than the American People. The Advisory Committee on Immunization Practices has also advised the Centers for Disease Control and Prevention (CDC) that girls as young as 9 years old be vaccinated. What is good for the Drug companies, in my opinion, is a crime against children. Like previous FDA frauds, the intent is to eventually make the vaccine mandatory. This will bring the greatest revenue for Merck from government-mandated regulations. The FDA's rationale is that Gardasil is most effective for young girls before they become sexually active. That expands the market even more. Gardasil is not cheap —$360 for a series of three shots. Not only is Gardasil completely worthless, like all other drugs, but also it has all the earmarks of causing as much devastation and horror as Vioxx, with a lot more profit!

The medical industry is sucking enough out of the American economy to cause the US not only to have to grovel for its daily bread, but to actually approach financial disaster. Besides that, it is turning a basically healthy population into one teeming with diseases. My hope is that the world will give more attention to observations made by one single individual who has no personal agenda, than by an industry whose annual sales are in the billions of dollars. An industry that gives millions of dollars to our elected officials. An industry, whose leaders are prepared to force their products on the American People by police and military enforcement, if necessary.

Now that the medical industry has succeeded in getting almost every senior citizen on a drug regimen, it has turned its greedy eyes to children. Even now, millions of children as young as infants are being drugged and vaccinated, not only in the United States, but all around the world. The elite drug pushers will always find an excuse to promote their products and they do not stop at the borders of the United States. Ritalin (a drug found to stunt growth and cause death) and other similar drugs are prescribed for children because they fidgeted, squirmed in their seat or were inattentive. Any excuse is imagined to push a drug. Today, millions of Canadian and US children are prescribed drugs for this "condition". Children in the foster care system, in particular, are being heavily poisoned. Some as young as three years old, are being screened for mental illnesses and started on psychiatric drugs for disorders such as schizophrenia, bipolar disorder and depression. This has the potential to label infants with psychiatric disorders while creating an endless market for psychiatric drugs and cause many diseases that will require more of their chemical solutions in the future. These children will be customers for life, short as their lives may be. Some drug companies are even marketing candy-flavored versions of these drugs. Sales of these drugs are now in the billions of dollars annually.

The drugging of children is obscene and draws attention to the lack of oversight that has been granted to drug companies by an under-educated public. The drugging of infants under the age of one is even more vile. As these children grow, they will be plagued with all sorts of disease that will seem to come for no apparent reason. Asthma is clearly traced to the early use of antibiotics. Reports of sudden deaths, strokes, heart attacks and hypertension in both children and adults taking drugs are spurring a new government study into medication's safety. But once again, a study can be made to achieve any desired results. Especially a government study, since the government, in my opinion, sometimes appears to be a branch of the pharmaceutical industry.

The US now has the highest infant mortality in the world. The doctors who are prescribing these drugs will have a lot to answer for. How long can we wait? I have traced many of the diseases we have in our society today for which there seems to be no explanation, such as asthma, birth tumors, allergies and many other disorders, to medicine, childhood vaccinations or mothers who were on medicine. I have seen evidence that children born to mothers who had been given antibiotics during pregnancy, had a higher than usual risk of developing Cerebral Palsy. Children are a great advertisement for the industry. Children, with their pristine immune systems, rebound, often easily and quickly from the most horrendous drug assaults made by the medical drug pushers.

Why is disease more prevalent in the older population? Because the older a person is, the more his immune system has been weakened by medicine. There are also other toxins in our society that are damaging to the human body, but medicine, because of its heavy and widespread use, is the great crippler.

America is now at the threshold of "Forced Medicine!"

Even today, it is not unheard of for parents to offer bribes to doctors to exempt their children from being vaccinated. Pet owners, who know the truth about "medicine," are paying veterinarians to exempt their pets from the violent assault known as "shots". Senior citizens may not be accepted by Senior Housing until their pet has had the "necessary" poisons ordered by the medical authorities. This is the power of an industry that has managed to infiltrate our government!

The medical industry stops at nothing to promote its products and to seize political power. Across this nation, an increasing number of persons are arrested at gunpoint, jailed, prosecuted and separated from their children by Child Protective Services. This is due to the demands of doctors who are so desperate to push their high-profit drug treatments onto patients, that they now resort to kidnapping children to override the parents choice of treatment. All this is done with the blessings of our elected officials. <u>Caution to all parents:</u> Look out! Social Services may be pounding on your door next when your physician disagrees with the decision you have made about the health care of your child.

There is some evidence that infant vaccinations including Vitamin K injections may be associated with leukemia. I have also found that the body does not readily utilize synthetic vitamins and minerals. I suggest that when in doubt, stay close to nature. It may be wise to avoid synthetic vitamins or synthetic anything.

Adults too, may soon be operated on, drugged and forced by law to undergo any medical procedure ordered by some doctor with a second opinion by his side. Through enormous political contributions, the drug companies have managed to so influence our Congress that it is intent on passing legislation favoring the medical industry. Forced medicine has been in the planning, and is about to arrive. The first step towards forced medicine is forced vaccinations. It is imperative that we say "No!" to forced vaccinations for ourselves, our children and even our household pets. With the advent of ObamaCare (socialized medicine) we have slid down that slippery slope! Pharmaceutical companies must be stopped now before it is too late. There should be no law that can force us to accept what we believe to be vile products or to accept statistics provided by those who have a vested interest in the sales, promotion or distribution of those products. I believe someone once said, "If we give up one freedom, we may soon lose them all." Those who tried to appease The Great Dictator confirmed this!

The medical industry now spends millions in its promotion of aspirin. They expect that millions will get them billions. I'm sure they are right. Did you know that every time you take aspirin you bleed a little into your gut? A microscope will show that the bowel movement of someone on daily aspirin has blood in it every time. If it is happening in your intestinal tract, it could easily be happening in your brain. It is a sorry thing, but the medical authorities have a habit of ignoring facts that do not suit their agenda. How many strokes are precipitated by chronic aspirin intake? How many fatal hemorrhages of the brain, spleen, liver, intestine, or lung occur after an automobile accident because the blood has been thinned with aspirin? The medical authorities are not counting. They don't want to know. An aspirin a day is as worthless as any other drug and possibly just as harmful. It will start you on the road to damage to the lining of your stomach, wheezing, breathlessness, ringing in the ears, hearing loss, chronic catarrh, runny nose, headache, confusion, nausea, vomiting, GI upset, GI bleeding, ulcers, rash, allergic reactions, hives, bruising, abnormal liver function tests, liver damage, and hepatitis. An aspirin a day guarantees one thing only: Future patients and future profits.

I've noticed that disease, death and medicine always walk hand in hand. One "perk" when famous is that everyone is made aware of the private circumstances surrounding a celebrity passing. Examples: Michael Jackson was on as many as 20 different medicines and surrounded by almost as many doctors. I remember how Elvis Presley died with all his medicines within reach; then Anna Nicole Smith, numerous medicines by her bedside. These are representative of millions of similar cases throughout our society. Wherever I find disease, I find medicine. When I find premature or unexpected death, I examine closely, and always there at patients bedside table were vials of medicine. Legal medicine which according to medical "studies" and "statistics" represented "giant strides" in the treatment of disease. One should consider that if it happens to a celebrity, it happens to ordinary unthinking folks as well.

When Frank Sinatra died, I was intent on examining his final scene. I had not heard that he had been a user of recreational drugs. I had heard that lately he had been suffering from several physical disorders. I wondered why. The answer came to me as no surprise. At the time of his death he was being drugged by his doctors to the tune of 100 pills of medicine a week. I did not find out how long this outrageous assault on his body had been taking place. These products are so toxic that even one pill must require prescription or supervision of a trained physician. Then how on earth was a man, gravely ill, who had constant bouts of pneumonia, kidney and bladder damage, Alzheimer-like symptoms, heart failure, cancer of the bladder, how could Frank Sinatra tolerate 17 poisons every day during what turned out to be the last days of his life and be expected to survive?

4. The President's Men

Our elected officials have played a great part in promoting the medical industry, partly because of their greed, and partly because of their fear to offend the hand that feeds them. The number of our representatives who appear to have sold us out to the drug industry is considerable. The highest officials in the land were not above greed and deal making. President Bush who had numerous direct ties to vaccine and drug manufacturers, spent more time and energy promoting the drug business than taking care of America's business. The drug industry had a combined lobbying and campaign contribution budget in 1999 and 2000 of almost $200 million dollars! Larger than any other industry, a large part of this was earmarked for President Bush. In return the president went beyond the call of duty. When the prospect of an Avian Flu outbreak was panicking people around the globe, President Bush had no intention of disappointing his benefactors. As President, he embarked on a plan to instill panic in this country by stating that as many as 2 million deaths in this country alone could arise from the bird flu. President Bush sent a letter to the Speaker of the House declaring it an "emergency" to seek congressional approval for $7 billion in order to respond to a "threat of avian and pandemic influenza."

Text of a Letter from the President to the Speaker of the House of Representatives

"Dear Mr. Speaker:

"Today, I outlined a strategy to address the threat of avian and pandemic influenza. This strategy is designed to meet three critical goals: to detect and contain outbreaks before they spread across the world, to protect the American people by stockpiling vaccines and antiviral drugs and accelerating the development of new vaccine technologies, and to ensure that Federal, State, and local communities are prepared for potential domestic outbreaks. To provide the necessary resources to immediately begin the implementation of this strategy, I ask the Congress to consider the enclosed requests, totaling $7.1 billion, for the Departments of Health and Human Services, Agriculture, Defense, Homeland Security, the Interior, State, and Veterans Affairs, as well as for International Assistance Programs.

"I hereby designate the proposals in the amount requested herein as emergency requirements, and I urge the Congress to act expeditiously on this request to ensure the country is prepared for this growing danger.

"The details of this request are set forth in the enclosed letter from the Director of the Office of Management and Budget."

Sincerely,

GEORGE W. BUSH

So the United States started out by placing an order for 20 million doses of a worthless drug (since all drugs are worthless) called Tamiflu, to treat an imaginary disease called the bird flu, a disease which existed only in the minds of the medical authorities and drug promoters, at a price of $100 per dose. That comes to a staggering $2 billion. As of now, so far as we know, on Planet Earth about 60 people have died of bird flu. All were involved in handling sick birds. There is, as of now, no recorded case of bird flu being transmitted from one human to another —something that is necessary before even an epidemic, much less a pandemic, could occur. I was surprised to turn up nothing to tie Bush to the profits produced by the product called Tamiflu.

After digging further, I found that Tamiflu was actually developed by a company called Gilead, of which Defense Secretary Donald Rumsfeld was made the chairman in 1997. Since Rumsfeld held major portions of stock in Gilead, he would profit to the tune of millions of dollars from the government's purchase of Tamiflu. It seems Bush and Rumsfeld had kept it all in the family. Bush actually killed two birds with one stone; and proved to be better suited for the drug business than the business of running the country. Once the deed was done and it was time for Rumsfeld to unload the Tamiflu stock, a private securities lawyer advised him that it was safer to hold on to the stock rather than sell and run the risk of being accused of trading on insider information.

The drug Tamiflu, completely worthless (like all other drugs) was stockpiled by countries around the world (the drug sales force has a long reach) to treat a disease that existed only in the minds of the drug promoters. The cost of these products, of course, went into the billions and billions of dollars. The drug industry is not only helping to destroy the economy of the US, but they are helping to bring the whole world to the threshold of financial ruin.

Tamiflu which proved, like most other drugs, to have dangerous side effects did not stop Japan from storing enough doses to treat 25 million people —another big sale for the Tamiflu makers! Behold the power of a pharmaceutical sales force with their political associates in Washington and around the world.

Rumsfeld has thus made millions of dollars on Tamiflu, assisted by the hyped avian flu threat, foreign leaders being brought into the fold and federal government contracts for his product. Rumsfeld is not the only political heavyweight benefiting from demand for Tamiflu. Former Secretary of State George Shultz, who was on Gilead's board, has sold more than $7 million worth of Gilead since the beginning of 2005. This is what has been uncovered so far. Remember, 90% of the pharmaceutical iceberg is under water!

There is no question that many of our elected representatives are unusually close to the pharmaceutical industry. Whether it is for the good of the American people or for their own selfish purposes remains to be seen. I am certain there are many deals being made; and these drug deals are very profitable for those involved; but costly to the American people and the people of the world. Note that when a handful of people die after being diagnosed with the Bird Flu, death is attributed to the Bird Flu. When thousands die after receiving the flu shot, death is rarely attributed to the flu shot. It would more than likely be attributed to "heart failure" or some pre-existing condition. The medical authorities not only have a foolproof system; their word has now become the law of the land, thanks to their cronies in the halls of Congress.

Our elected officials are certainly aware of what is going on. I have found that without question some of our highest-ranking officials, who have not been able to contribute anything to the solution of the economic and health care problems of American Society, have proven very proficient in promoting the products of the pharmaceutical industry. Bush had a great idea that certainly must have pleased his friends in the drug industry. His plan would most likely have included forcing pharmaceutical products on the American people. President George W. Bush actually asked Congress to consider giving him powers to use the military to enforce quarantines in case of an avian influenza epidemic. Of course, the ones who would decide if there were an epidemic would be the medical authorities. This includes those who would profit from the sale of the drugs that the government would have to purchase in the event of an epidemic. It would be interesting to observe the thought process that prompted President Bush to promote an industry that was draining from the American economy more than a trillion dollars a year.

In January 2006, the FDA announced the Bush administration's latest gift to Big Pharma in a statement that said people who believe they have been injured by drugs approved by the FDA should not be allowed to sue drug companies in state courts. These damages would be so great so as to be ruinous to the drug companies. The plan was to save the drug companies by having the American people foot the bill.

There have been many bogus alarms such as the earlier swine flu scare (1973) that gave Congress an excuse to immunize companies from all liability for the hastily prepared swine flu vaccine that ended up doing nothing but brain-damaging many Americans and causing a progressive multiple sclerosis-like disease.

Swine-Flu Bribe Fever!

Posted: December 07, 2009

9:53 pm Eastern

By Chelsea Schilling

© 2009 WorldNetDaily

"World Health Organization scientists are suspected of accepting secret bribes from vaccine manufacturers to influence the U.N. Organization's H1N1 pandemic declaration, according to Danish and Swedish newspapers. Meanwhile, pharmaceutical profits from Swine Flu related drugs have soared —with earnings between $10 billion and $15 billion in 2009, investment bank JP Morgan estimates. As WND (WorldNetDaily) reported, the WHO Director General Margaret Chan initially raised the influenza pandemic alert to its second highest level in May —but evidence reveals the agency may have made it easier to classify the flu outbreak as a pandemic by changing its definition to omit 'enormous

numbers of deaths and illness' just prior to making its declaration.

"The world was gripped with fears of Swine Flu as the alert increased from Phase 5 to Phase 6, the highest level. Immediately, pharmaceutical companies began working to develop vaccines, and countries tailored their responses to address the situation."

President Bush pushed drugs even in his farewell speech. He talked about the medicine that was giving AIDS patients longer life. My own study, small as it may have been, found that medicine was shortening the lives of AIDS patients! I investigated and interviewed many AIDS patients and found that those who rejected the medicine (AZT at that time) were the longest living survivors of the disease. There was great evidence that if AIDS were curable, and I feel certain that it is curable, drugs will never play a part in that cure.

As for President Bush and Don Rumsfeld, they proved to have done a much better job promoting their pharmaceutical interests than promoting the interest of this country. Senator Obama was not to be left out of the Drug bonanza. Barack Obama bought shares in Baxter, the company many say is responsible for the H1N1 swine flu pandemic. (This is according to Infowars Ireland 11/18/09). He also bought shares in AVI BioPharma, a drug company working to develop a medicine to treat avian flu victims. Right after he bought the shares and still a senator at that time, Obama introduced the first comprehensive bill to address the threat of avian influenza pandemic —AVIAN Act (S.969) Then Sen. Obama began pushing for an increase in federal financing to fight Avian Flu, a move that eventually helped lead to the Senate's approval of a $3.8 billion appropriation to fight the flu. The author of this book, as did many other Americans, endorsed, supported and voted for Barack Obama; but this is not the "change" that we had in mind.

Another example of the many politicians who have been found to be on the receiving end of health care industry benefits is Senator Bill Frist, who, unbelievably to this day holds a position of prominence in American politics.

THE FOUNDATION FOR TAXPAYER AND CONSUMER RIGHTS

Sept. 21, 2005

Director, Division of Enforcement

U.S. Securities and Exchange Commission

100 F Street NE

Washington, D.C. 20549-0213

"Ms. Thomsen:

"We are writing to request that you investigate insider-trading activity between Thomas Frist, Jr. and his brother Bill Frist, the current U.S. Senate Majority Leader. Thomas Frist, Jr., the largest individual shareholder in Hospital Corporation of America (HCA), with 5.5 million shares that were worth over $263 million at the end of trading today. Mr. Frist is an HCA Director, and has also held the positions of Chairman, President and Chief Executive Officer at the company.

"Senator Frist sold all the HCA shares owned by himself and his immediate family, worth millions of dollars according to U.S. Senate disclosures, just two weeks prior to a disappointing earnings report that resulted in a double digit drop in the value of the shares.

"Frist's father founded the company. His brother, Thomas, ran the company and continues to hold a position of influence. Thomas Frist, Jr. qualifies as an insider under the Securities and Exchange Act.

"Senator Frist instructed the manager of his shares to sell them in mid-June as the price of HCA stock was peaking. His shares were sold by July 1 and his family's shares sold on July 8. The company's stock value fell precipitously on July 13 after the announcement of poor quarterly earnings that failed to meet expectations.

"Given the close relationship between Senator Frist and Thomas Frist, it is imperative that their communications concerning the sale of Senator Frist's HCA stock be investigated fully including use of your subpoena power to acquire phone and financial records, board meeting minutes, and other pertinent records to verify the veracity of the assertions by the subjects of the investigation."

Sincerely,

Jamie Court Carmen Balber

cc Eliot Spitzer, New York State Attorney General

U.S. Attorneys, Southern District of New York, Southern District of Tennessee

Here are two more revealing articles about the Frist fiasco

Dr. Frist Immunizes Big Pharma

By Dan Hamburg/Executive Director, Voice of the Environment

Monday, January 23rd, 2006

"Hidden in the folds of the thickly pork-laden Department of Defense Appropriations bill that slid through Congress just before Christmas and was signed into law a day before New Year's was a big slab of holiday cheer for the pharmaceutical industry. There were no press releases from congressional offices and no mention in the news —maybe no one wanted to take credit for this latest assault on the 14th amendment.

"The so-called "Frist provision" —named after the ethically challenged physician-turned-politician Bill Frist —will immunize Big Pharma from responsibility for vaccine-related injuries. The main rationale for this latest gift to industry at the expense of the public is —you may have guessed it —the War on Terror! Our representatives in Congress pled that corporations like Merck, GlaxoSmithKline, Wyeth, and Eli Lilly might just have to close up shop if they were forced to take responsibility for injuries caused by their products."
—(Dan Hamburg is a former member of Congress).

Robert F. Kennedy Jr. investigates the government cover-up of a mercury/autism scandal.

"Senate Majority Leader Bill Frist, who has received $873,000 in contributions from the pharmaceutical

industry, has been working to immunize vaccine makers from liability in 4,200 lawsuits that have been filed by the parents of injured children. On five separate occasions, Frist has tried to seal all of the government's vaccine-related documents —including the Simpsonwood transcripts —and shield Eli Lilly, the developer of thimerosal, from subpoenas. In 2002, the day after Frist quietly slipped a rider known as the "Eli Lilly Protection Act" into a homeland security bill, the company contributed $10,000 to his campaign and bought 5,000 copies of his book on bioterrorism, "Deadly Immunity." —Rolling Stone, Jun 20, 2005

Pharma Pays to Sway Congress

Jim Drinkard, USA TODAY

(Excerpts)

"When Sen. Bill Frist needed help in November for a quick tour celebrating the victories of newly elected Republican senators, he did not have to look far. A Gulfstream corporate jet owned by drugmaker Schering-Plough was ready to zip the Senate majority leader to stops in Florida, Georgia and the Carolinas".

"The drug companies' corporate planes have been made available not only to Frist, but also for dozens of trips taken by other powerful lawmakers. House Speaker Dennis Hastert, R-Ill., took at least four trips to GOP fundraising events in the past two years aboard Pfizer's Gulfstream.

"Drug companies and their officials contributed at least $17million to federal candidates in last year's elections, including nearly $1 million to President Bush and more

than $500,000 to his opponent, John Kerry. At least 18 members of Congress received more than $100,000 apiece."

"Frist isn't the senator from Tennessee —he's the senator from the state of Health Care Industry Influence —he's gotten more than $2 million from the health-care sector, giving him the dubious distinction of raising more cash from health-care interests than 98 percent of his colleagues," says Nick Nyhart, executive director of Public Campaign.

"The pharmaceutical industry has spent more than $800 million in lobbying and campaign contributions since 1998.", according to the Center for Public Integrity, a watchdog group. —Andrea Stone, USA Today.

We have been deceived and we continue to be deceived by our elected officials including the president, himself. The courts have recently ruled natural healing to be illegal. The brainwashed populace remains silent and submissive. The rest of us have to fight with nothing but our voice and the voices of the millions of people who have been damaged by medicine: the voices of the millions, who's children have been damaged or killed by these vile products; and we have to win this fight in spite of the great cover-up by the thousands and thousands of death certificates that read, *"died from heart failure".*

It is interesting to note the tremendous reach of the drug promoters.

Updated Fri. Nov. 23, 2007 10:26 AM ET, from the Associated Press:

"LONDON — The British government unveiled plans Thursday to provide vaccinations for the entire population in the advent of a flu pandemic."

What a sale! Big Pharma strikes again!

Does an agency like the FDA have a mind of its own, or is it controlled by the medical industry and special interests? To answer, consider the story of aspartame and how Donald Rumsfeld manipulated FDA to put a carcinogenic neurotoxin on the market, one for which FDA had repeatedly denied approval since it causes brain tumors.

Rumsfeld was CEO of the G. D. Searle Co., producer of

aspartame/NutraSweet/Equal. FDA would not approve Searle's chemical sweetener plainly because it is undeniably toxic, releases methyl alcohol (as in rotgut booze) then converts into formaldehyde, formic acid and diketopiperazine. Deadly, deadly, deadly!

So what to do? Dangerous Donald had political clout as part of newly elected Ronald Reagan's transition team. So the night of Reagan's inauguration the FDA Commissioner who had stood in the way of aspartame approval was fired. A new stooge, Arthur Hayes, was appointed to run the Food and Drug Administration, which was then effectively decapitated. The now ousted Commissioner Dr. Jere Goyan was about to sign revocation of aspartame into law, but he received a call from the Reagan team at 3:00 AM demanding his resignation. Next Reagan signed an executive order that made FDA powerless to act on aspartame until

Hayes got to Washington to take over. Hayes over-ruled FDA's scientific Board of Inquiry, which refused to approve aspartame because of brain tumors and general toxicity.

Aspartame is now sold as NutraSweet, Equal, Spoonful, E951, Canderel and Benevia, and is in such popular products as Diet Coke, Diet Pepsi, Diet Snapple and Sugar Free Kool-Aid. Hundreds of millions consume it worldwide. It is in prescription and over-the-counter drugs and, believe it or not, <u>Aspartame is added to products sold to treat the problems it causes.</u> It is in pediatric drugs and vitamins with consequent devastations to our children and youth.

If you are using Aspartame, and suffer from fibromyalgia symptoms, cancer, spasms, shooting pains, joint pain, seizures, memory loss, numbness in your legs, cramps, vertigo, dizziness, headaches, tinnitus, joint pain, depression, anxiety attacks, slurred speech, or blurred vision—you may have ASPARTAME DISEASE! It also can precipitate diabetes, simulates and aggravates diabetic retinopathy and neuropathy, destroys the optic nerve, causes diabetics to go into convulsions and even interacts with insulin. It should be noted Splenda/sucralose is a chlorocarbon poison that is very dangerous for diabetics. A new safe sweetener with no additives is called Just Like Sugar which is usually available in places like Whole Foods.

Dr. Betty Martini, D. Hum. Lectured for the

World Environmental Conference in 1995

In 1998 a post Dr. Martini wrote to a neurological list was plagiarized and sent out in mass by a "Nancy Markle." A networker put it on hundreds of international networks, so it made world news. MS victims were walking out of wheelchairs; symptoms on the FDA list of 92 symptoms were vanishing as sick people on aspartame returned to normal health. Such things as headaches, joint pain, vision problems, seizures and male sexual dysfunction simply ceased with elimination. Cori Brackett, one of the MS victims who walked out of her wheelchair, was co-founder of Sound and Fury Productions. She produced the documentary, "Sweet Misery: A Poisoned World." —www.soundandfury.tv

So powerful has consumer protest against aspartame been that the largest maker of aspartame in Europe, Holland Sweetener, quit making it in 2006 and in America in January 2009, Merisant went bankrupt for 230 million dollars. Aspartame is in the toilet and consumers are flushing it!

Also Dr. H. J. Roberts, M.D. in 2001 released the 1000 page medical text, Aspartame Disease: An Ignored Epidemic, www.sunsentpress.com giving the mechanism by which aspartame can precipitate MS. The text is filled with all the medical problems she lectured on at the World Environmental Conference. Monsanto who owned NutraSweet at the time could not put out the fire and sold the company. Finally the word got around the globe so Ajinomoto who now owns most of the aspartame industry said they were changing the name from aspartame to AminoSweet! Be warned.

You can reach Dr. Martini at bettym19@mindspring.com

Rumsfeld and Bush may not have served the country too well; but they were heroes to the pharmaceutical industry. It is important to observe that these two were far from being alone in their pharmaceutical endeavors.

Bush's allegiance to the drug industry was obvious. When the Anthrax vaccine proved harmful to our fighting men, the Bush administration argued that the US military should resume mandatory Anthrax vaccinations of its personnel. Where did he get his medical expertise? Probably from the pharmaceutical lobbyists who were ever ready with their "political contributions". We then find former high-ranking health officials with close ties to the Bush administration helping a Michigan-based pharmaceutical company secure multi-million dollar federal contracts for the purchase of the Anthrax vaccine.

PENTAGON HID TRUTH ON ANTHRAX VACCINE

Friday, January 06, 2006 - FreeMarketNews.com

"Over the last seven years, the Pentagon only revealed information about a small fraction of the cases in which serious complications caused by giving soldiers the anthrax vaccine, according to the Daily Press. The Pentagon had repeatedly promised to send Congress reports anytime a soldier was hospitalized after taking the vaccine from 1998 to 2000.

"In the last seven years, 1.2 million soldiers have been forced to take the anthrax vaccine. Less than 100 cases of complications from the vaccine were reported to Congress, leading experts to project that about one

in 100,000 would suffer from severe complications after taking the vaccine. However documents recently obtained by the Daily Press show that over 20,000 soldiers were hospitalized after being subjected to the shot. Among the severe complications that were not reported were three cases of Lou Gehrig's disease, a disease that kills the muscles and nerves in the body and always leads to death."

In a two-year span, the nation's only licensed Anthrax vaccine maker went from pleading poverty to announcing $100 million in acquisitions, including other pharmaceutical companies and a new manufacturing plant near Washington, D.C

President Bush's request that every service member in the Armed Forces must be given the Anthrax vaccine was followed by a group of soldiers suing the government to avoid being forced to take this horrendous product. What a shameful irony that hundreds of thousands of US troops were told that even though they are fighting for freedom, they could soon face Court Martial for refusing to take a vaccine that has led to disabilities, chronic illnesses and even death to others. After hundreds of reported illnesses and several thousand more queries about potential diseases and disorders caused by this product, the Defense Department started allowing troops deployed overseas to opt out of receiving the Anthrax vaccine without penalty. The government sometimes backs down from its efforts to accommodate the drug industry, but not often, not easily, and not willingly.

President Bush had big plans!

Stockpile Would Permit Mass Inoculations

By Justin Gillis

Washington Post Staff Writer

(Excerpt)

Friday, March 12, 2004

"The government is preparing to buy enough experimental anthrax vaccine for 25 million people, a stockpile that would permit mass inoculations in numerous U.S. cities if terrorists launched a broad assault with the deadly germ.

"The new vaccine would be the most significant addition to the national anti-terrorism stockpile since the Bush administration fulfilled a pledge to buy enough smallpox vaccine for every citizen of the United States."

We have already given up our first freedom. We allowed our children to be vaccinated by force. Next, we allowed our household pets in the name of health to become victims of these people and their products. The Rabies vaccine is a good example. Worthless as all the others, it has caused much disease and suffering to our pets. Why is the Rabies vaccine deemed so necessary, simply because the doctor and drug lobbies says so. I found it, like all the others, to be not only worthless but also harmful. First the children. Then our pets. Next in line, our fighting men were subjected to medicine by force. The next step, we, ourselves will be taken by a doctor with a court order in one hand and a police escort at their side to a place of medical procedure and we may be operated on, electro-shocked or whatever is the whim of the medical authority. The people of America are approaching a slippery slope. It is urgent that we stop short in our tracks and wake up to what is going on around us.

Many congressmen will give their allegiance to the medical industry in spite of their sworn service to the American people. The list is long. The apparent sellouts are too numerous to mention. Visit the list of contributors and political contributions. $100,000 contributions are not uncommon. Contributions of this size are not usually made simply because of admiration of the politician. The health care industry always backs the winners. How do they manage this? It is very simple. All political contributions by the medical industry to our elected officials would be too numerous to mention; but these few are especially worthy of notice:

Al Gore —$100,000

Joe Lieberman —$100,000

Rudolph Giuliani —$98,000

Senator Obama —$150,000

Senator Hillary Clinton —$140,000

Governor Mitt Romney —$100,000

Mayor Rudy Giuliani —$90,000

Senator Chris Dodd —$70,000

The above mentioned are the tip of the iceberg. A review, for instance, of Lieberman's campaign finance reports by the nonpartisan Center for Responsive Politics shows health professionals and the insurance industry have contributed millions to his campaigns.

Insurance, health care firms give Lieberman big bucks

By Bill Cummings, Investigative Reporter/Danbury News Times

Published: 08:55 p.m., Saturday, December 19, 2009

(Excerpts)

"U.S. Sen. Joe Lieberman has taken in millions of dollars in campaign contributions from the insurance and health industry he's now accused of protecting from meaningful health care reform.

"A review of Lieberman's campaign finance reports by the nonpartisan Center for Responsive Politics shows health professionals and the insurance industry have contributed more than $2.1 million to his campaigns since 1989.

"The Connecticut senator has raised about $49 million overall, including millions from financial firms, lawyers, real estate interests and pro-Israeli groups."

"Campaign records show contributions from health and insurance interests spiked in 2006 after the senator lost the Democratic primary and ran as an Independent Democrat. Lieberman collected more than $20 million during the 2006 election cycle, almost half his lifetime total, and beat Democrat Ned Lamont and Republican Alan Schlesinger."

"Among Lieberman's biggest lifetime contributors is indeed the Hartford-based Aetna insurance company, which has contributed $112,618 through political action committees and individuals. The Travelers Companies, also based in Hartford, has contributed $72,119.

"Purdue Pharma, a Stamford pharmaceutical company, contributed $150,100 to Lieberman through individuals and PACs, making it the senator's fourth-largest single contributor.

"Pharmaceutical giant Pfizer Inc. contributed $85,000 through individuals and PACs.

"Reports on file with the Federal Election Commission show Lieberman accepted tens of thousands of dollars from PACs representing nurses, doctors, hospitals, chemists, ambulance firms, dermatologists and medical associates —just about anyone associated with the health care industry.

"Money also flowed from PACs representing insurance companies such as Blue Cross Blue Shield, Anthem, CIGNA, Health Net and UnitedHealth."

"In a 2004 report, the nonpartisan Center for Public Integrity quoted an insurance industry representative as saying Lieberman was widely recognized as the "go-to guy on the Democratic side of the aisle.

"The center's report noted Pfizer had long been a Lieberman contributor and offered examples of how the senator introduced legislation that benefited the company.

"For example, the center found that between 1998 and 2003, Lieberman cosponsored nine bills Pfizer had directly lobbied for, varying from tax breaks to patent extensions.

"In the 2002 election cycle, more than 70 percent of Pfizer's money went to GOP candidates. But Lieberman was an exception, the center reported. During that period,

the company increased its donations to Lieberman even though he was not up for re-election."

Investigative reporter Bill Cummings can be reached at bcummings@ctpost.com. Information from the Los Angeles Times was included in this story.

As might be expected, Lieberman voted full immunity for the pharmaceutical companies.

Lieberman the Moralist

When Clinton couldn't muster an apology for his behavior in the Monica Lewinsky affair, Lieberman gave him a public push from the floor of the Senate that captured headlines. Clinton's behavior was "immoral," "harmful" and "compromised his moral authority," Lieberman declared at a time when other Democrats were silent or toeing the party line. —John Solomon Associated Press

Separate analyses by the Center for Responsive Politics, and by The New York Times show that Senator Clinton has received $854,462 from the health care industry in 2005-6, a larger amount than any candidate except Senator Santorum, with $977,354. Interesting to note that during her 2000 Senate campaign, she sharply criticized her opponent, Rick A. Lazio, as being beholden to the pharmaceutical industry for taking donations from drugmakers.

These contributions are greatly overshadowed by those given to George Bush. Bush appears to have been the drug industry's archangel. The fact that the drug industry plays both ends against the middle guarantees that they will be backing the winner, whoever he or she is. The losers are the American People and the people of the world.

Quote

"We must ensure the federal government acts as a partner with the private sector, providing the incentives and protections necessary to bring more and better drugs and vaccines to market faster." —Sen. Richard Burr, R-N.C. 2003-2004. Richard Burr received donations from the Health industry amounting to over $500,000.

38 Senators With Up to $13.4 Million in Pharmaceutical Stock

Approve Drug Industry's Sweetheart Deal

(Excerpt)

SANTA MONICA, Calif., 12/22/2005 /U.S. Newswire/ —"38 U.S. Senators with up to $13.4 million in pharmaceutical holdings increased the value of their stock portfolios last night when they approved an amendment to the defense *appropriations bill that immunizes drug makers from accountability to the public when they sell dangerous drugs and other products, according to the Foundation for Taxpayer and Consumer Rights (FTCR).*

"When Senators can vote to harm the health and safety of the American public and line their own pockets while they're at it, the motive behind every vote is in question. No Senator should be able to vote in his own financial interests at the expense of the public," said *Carmen Balber, consumer advocate with the nonprofit, nonpartisan Foundation for Taxpayer and Consumer Rights.*

"FTCR released an analysis of Senate personal financial disclosures last week, revealing that 42 senators — 27 Republicans and 15 Democrats —held pharmaceutical stock worth between $8.1 and $16 million in 2004. Senators earned an additional $2.5 to $7.2 million in capital gains and dividends, and two senators' spouses also earned salaries from pharmaceuticals."

"The 38 Senators with pharmaceutical stock that voted for the provision are: Allen (R-Virginia.)

Bayh (D-Indiana.)

Bingaman (D-New Mexico)

Bond (R-Missouri)

Boxer (D-California)

Brownback (R-Kansas)

Burns (R-Montana)

Carper (D-Delaware)

Coburn (R-Oklahoma)

Cochran (R-Mississippi)

Conrad (D-North Dakota)

Crapo (R-Idaho)

Dayton (D-Minnesota)

DeWine (R-Ohio)

Dole (R-North Carolina)

Ensign (R-Nevada)

Feinstein (D-California)

Frist (R-Tennessee)

Hatch (R-Utah)

Hutchison (R-Texas)

Inhofe (R-Oklahoma)

Isakson (R-Georgia)

Kerry (D-Massachusetts)

Kyl (R-Arizona)

Landrieu (D-Louisiana)

Lautenberg (D-New Jersey)

Levin (D-Michigan)

Lieberman (D-Connecticut)

Lott (R-Mississippi)

Reed (D-Rhode Island)

Reid (D-Nevada)

Roberts (R-Kansas)

Stevens (R-Alaska)

Sununu (R-New Hampshire)

Talent (R-Missouri)

Vitter (R-Louisiana)

Voinovich (R-Ohio)

Warner (R-Virginia)

Four Senators with pharmaceutical holdings did not vote."

It seems to me that decent people do not run for public office. If they do, they become tainted once they get there. I do not have a complete list of the members of Congress that appear to have sold us out to the medical establishment, but the names go on and on. I am forced to believe that if an elected official were in any way to expose or reveal the truth about the pharmaceutical industry and its intimacy with our public officials, he or she would become an outcast. I feel the same way about the medical industry: An honest doctor would not be tolerated.

I have found from my small study that covers more than 50 years of investigation, observation, and even self-experimentation that the use of drugs and vaccines in the treatment and prevention of disease is one great fraud!

Doctors sit back comfortably while Americans worry about being able to afford their health care. I have found that those who can afford it are no better off than those who cannot. Americans are not getting much health from the health care providers. Americans are sick. I find very few people who are well. The fact is the medical industry is not in the business of making us well. They are in the business of selling us drugs, surgeries and other medical products and procedures. We are born basically with good health —that is nature's intent —but the medical experts seem to have other plans for us.

Whenever I look at people who make up governmental, hospital and medical health advisory boards, I find financial ties to pharmaceutical companies. Emergency-room services are necessary, helpful and have saved lives; but the Medical Industry has become so bloated that between the millions of unnecessary operations and the drugging of everyone in sight, they produce their own diseases and guarantee for themselves an endless supply of future patients.

The American Dream has changed.

Organized medicine has seen to that:

You will develop an illness;

You will start taking drugs;

You will start taking more drugs to counter the effects of the previous drugs;

You will be admitted to the hospital;

You will undergo surgeries;

You will die slowly, painfully and without dignity after your life savings have been completely wiped out.

If this is the agenda of the medical industry, it is working fine. They're doing a great job!

All that is necessary for our well being is the immune system in all its glory be encouraged, and more importantly, unhampered in its God-given and pre-ordained ability to protect our health and to cure just about every disease under the sun.

The medical industry has found that there is no business like show business and they have put on a great exhibition: Tubes, stethoscopes, scanners, doctors, nurses, charts, syringes, long white hallways, great buildings and clean linen. And multi-million dollar machines for detecting diseases. Diseases for which they have found no cure! Broadway itself could have not put on a better show.

When medical studies admit that some drugs may be harmful, they are simply clouding the issue. The fact is that all drugs are harmful. All drugs are poisonous. The American people are being brainwashed, duped and poisoned all at the same time.

When someone asks, "What should we do when we have a disease?" Should we do nothing?" The answer is usually "Yes!" Do nothing and allow the power of the immune system to do its pre-ordained work unhampered. That implies bringing the body and bloodstream back as close as possible to its original pristine condition and cleaning out of the veins and arteries the morbid matter, often the residue of medicinal drugs that have been allowed to accumulate there. The human body is a self-healing and self-cleansing entity. In our society we have a tendency to pollute the body with an overuse of acidic foods and products, such as coffee, alcohol, meat, sugar, chemicals and of course, medicine. Alkalinity is the means of bringing health to a sick body. To reduce to a bare minimum all acidic foods and substances, such as aspartame, coffee, alcohol, drugs, chemicals and medicine; and allow the immune system to rejuvenate and perform its basic function. The basic function of the immune system is to protect and defend the body against all disease and disorders; and it will work miracles if it is allowed to do this.

Not only have we, the people of America rewarded failure; we have prostrated ourselves before it. We have allowed ourselves to be poisoned in the name of health. We have worshipped the Golden Calf of Medicine. We have fallen to our knees before the grand buildings of Medical America. The thick floor coverings, the shiny nameplates, the fabulous panorama of the great medical societies have blinded us like tinsel to a child. So adamant are we, the American people, in seeking an easy way to compensate for a self-indulgent lifestyle that we have knelt before the paper dragon of medicine. A monster that has the ability to produce every disease known to man; but not the capability of curing even one of those diseases, not even the common cold!

I don't know how far back the shame of the American medical industry goes; but 100 years ago, the daring Dr. Henry Lindlahr, who founded one of the early cancer research clinics in America discovered, by experimentation, that irritation of a tumor would cause it to become cancerous. This was the first cancer breakthrough that I could find in recorded history. This finding was rejected. Lindlahr was shunned by his colleagues. As far as the medical authorities were concerned, his research was null and void. Of course his findings were unacceptable because the authorities did not approve of the results. The fact is it just didn't suit their agenda. The same scenario repeats itself today. Not one vaccine has ever prevented anything. Not one drug has ever cured anything. Yet the search goes on for drugs and vaccines. The medical experts will not back down. They are going to find something to sell, and they are going to sell it no matter what; and by force, if necessary. The next move is up to the American People.

The fact is that orthodoxy in science in general has historically followed this closed-minded path for centuries. Nearly all discoveries are by independents who are summarily shunned until decades or even centuries later they are finally recognized for their achievements. And until then, humanity remains unnecessarily poorer because of political correctness. This sorryful condition is just as prevalent today as it has been for centuries. It will remain so until personal greed can no longer be rewarded.

If the Bush's and Rumsfeld's of our political society were to stop pushing worthless and harmful medical products, and tend instead to the business of serving their constituents; if they were to divest themselves of medical stocks, if they refused donations or gifts from the medical industry, we might, at the very least, be able to solve America's economic problems. The first and foremost problem being the trillion dollar a year health care bill created by an industry that receives no oversight, that has no transparency, that is allowed to police itself and that through less than honorable means has now become the law of the land. If we had stopped this unholy situation ten years ago, America today would be debt-free. America would no longer be a burden to itself and to the world. We could support those among us who are tired or weary, who have had more than a normal amount of work thrust upon them and require some welfare or recreation. We could support aliens, legal or otherwise. These are not the culprits. These are the people we referred to when we said, "Bring me your poor!"

But now we are the poor. We have been made poor by an industry with no conscience and by elected officials with no scruples and by a populace that has been brainwashed by medical advertising. Advertising that contains no message and is done with the sole purpose of brainwashing. Americans are in a stupor. They are dazed and beaten by a giant parasite that gives with one hand and destroys with the other. The Medical Industry must be made transparent, it must be admonished and it must be toppled. It must undergo a metamorphosis so great as to become unrecognizable, unrecognizable but beautiful! Every business has a gray area; but this industry has grown too gray. It has grown too powerful for its own good or ours. The time has come to say "No!" to the Medical Industry. The time has come to say "No!" to Medical Power. The time has come to say "Yes!" to American Freedom!

We may never be privy to all the deals that have been made between members of Congress and the pharmaceutical industry. We may never know how the US Health care bill rose to over a trillion dollars a year and we will never forget the pain that comes to the average American who, in spite of being a citizen of the greatest and wealthiest nation on earth, must bear the pain and shame of a $10 trillion budget deficit that continues to grow out of control. This nation has been hit hard; but nothing will be worse than forced medicine now in the planning stages for the American people as well as the people of the world. How the oncoming holocaust of forced medicine can be achieved is elementary. Just ask Governor Rick Perry.

He has ties to Merck and orders mandatory vaccinations. He says that it is just a coincidence that he and eight other lawmakers received donations of $5,000 each from Merck lobbyists just a few days before mandating the drug giant's HPV cervical cancer vaccine for all females in Texas ages 12 and up. Perry has several ties to Merck and Women in Government. One of the drug company's three lobbyists in Texas is Mike Toomey, Governor Perry's former chief of staff. Perry's current chief of staff's mother-in-law, Texas Republican State Representative Dianne White Delisi, is a state director for Women in Government.

"Our new report shows that great progress is being made in the fight against cervical cancer," said Mary Brooks Beatty, President of Women In Government. *"However, this disease is almost completely preventable and we need to ensure that all women have access to the most appropriate cervical cancer prevention technologies, that socioeconomic status is not a barrier to receiving care, and that women around the world benefit from the tools that have helped make a difference in the battle against cervical cancer in the United States."*

Many of the bills introduced so far to make the shot mandatory have been introduced by members of a bi-partisan women's state legislators group called Women In Government. Further investigation finds that Women in Government's website lists the following drug companies as donors: 3M Pharmaceuticals, Abbott, Adeza Biomedical, Allergan, Inc., Amgen, AstraZeneca Pharmaceuticals, Bayer HealthCare, Boehringer Ingelheim Pharmaceuticals, Inc., Bristol-Myers Squibb Company, Bristol-Myers Squibb Foundation, Catalis, Digene Corporation, Eli Lilly and Company, GlaxoSmithKline, Hoffmann-LaRoche, Inc., Johnson & Johnson, Merck & Company, Inc., Novartis Pharmaceuticals, Novo Nordisk, Inc., Pfizer, Inc., PhRMA, Sanofi Aventis, Schering-Plough Corporation, Solvay Pharmaceuticals, Inc., and Wyeth Pharmaceuticals.

It is time that balance is restored. We must take the good of medicine because there is some good; but we must do away with what is wrong! This can be accomplished simply by applying oversight and transparency. We must tear away the veil of secrecy that surrounds the Congress of the United States and the Health Care Industry. We can no longer be polite. The time has come for rudeness. The time has come for action. The time has come for a fight to the finish if necessary!

This outrageous industry has infiltrated Congress, our schools, such groups as "Women in Government", our colleges, the media, even the courts have been brought into the fold. By excessive and sophisticated means of brainwashing, without ever having cured one disease, they have convinced the entire population of America and of the world, that the prevention or curing of diseases of the elderly, our children, newborn infants, even our household pets, requires the intake or injection of a toxic substance created by them, manufactured by themselves, promoted and sold by they, themselves. They now have the audacity to demand that these products be thrust upon the people of America and of the world by government mandate and physical force, if necessary!

5. Cancer

Cancer is a disease caused by great irritation or assault, usually to the bloodstream, and caused usually by medicinal drugs. Radiation from CT Scans, X-Rays, Mammograms are also high on the list of causes. Pre-cancerous conditions, such as cysts, moles, tumors and other abnormalities can become malignant from irritation, biopsy and sometimes by surgical removal. These procedures are often called routine medical procedures, and often, they are the beginning of the end for the patient.

The cure for most cancer is simply to eliminate the cause and create an alkaline environment within the body where out of control cancer cells cannot survive. Anything that depresses the immune system, such as over indulgence in acidic foods, obesity, or invasive or harmful products or procedures can be cancer causing. The ability of the immune system to cure the disease is sometimes so powerful that the cancer is defeated not because of drug or medical intervention, but in spite of it. The medical authorities insist that the cure comes as a packaged product or medical procedure, and for that reason they have gone 100 years without finding a cure. The fact is that cancer can never be cured by drugs. It is caused by drugs. The main cure for this disease is removal of the cause combined with the natural healing ability of the human body while being enhanced by an alkaline diet.

The first cancer breakthrough came 100 years ago when Dr. Henry Lindlahr found that biopsy of a tumor would cause that tumor to become cancerous. Not only were his findings displeasing to the medical authorities, the findings were rejected and the doctor became an outcast. Today, in complete disregard to these findings, the medical authorities continue the practice of tumor biopsy. The industry is not only causing most of the cancer in our society with medicinal drugs, radiation and surgery; but is causing even more devastation with its testing and other treatments.

When the doctor says, "there is no cure..." such as in "there is no cure for pancreatic cancer", this is simply another one of those tricks at which these people excel. The fact is they cannot cure anything. Not so long as their business is not in curing, but rather in the sales and promotion of drugs and other medical products and procedures. Yet, the fact remains that there is a cure. Patients with the most serious cancers are often given five years to live by the doctors, which is usually an accurate estimate, since the patient is about to be poisoned with drugs. I myself have discovered that the cure for the worst cases of cancer may take about the same length of time.

The cure is simply to remove the cause, which can be the overuse of acidic foods, acidic products, chemicals, toxins, but more than often, it is medicinal drugs. The patient then embarks on a holistic lifestyle that includes a mainly alkaline diet creating an environment within his or her body where tumors cannot thrive and are sent into remission. Except in final stages of a disease, the patient can recover completely in about five years. It is a long slow process; but recovery in five years is preferable to death in five years, except to those who are in the business of promoting medicine. Death, when it occurs in a cancer patient, will be recorded as due to cancer, but drugs cause the weakening of the immune system that allowed the disease to flourish.

When the doctor says that cancer is curable if caught early, that is true. The immune system is more successful in dealing with cancer in its early stages than in its advanced stages. The fact is, that the doctor has nothing to do with the cure. He is usually the cause of the cancer's advancement. The first symptom of the disease is often a tumor, which the body can deal with successfully when allowed and encouraged to do so without interference from drugs, surgery or biopsy. The first step in the treatment of cancer should be the removal of the cause. In our western industrialized culture, there are many causes, but it is usually medicinal drugs. For the doctor to stand by while a tumor goes into remission might be sufficient for the physician to receive credit for the cure; but what often happens is that a benign tumor is biopsied. This causes the tumor to turn cancerous. Then the patient is given chemotherapy that can damage the immune system, often to such a degree that cancer becomes a disease of the entire bloodstream.

The doctor is never responsible for the cure of cancer unless he or she allows the immune system to do its pre-ordained work. This of course, is not allowed in the practice of medicine. The practice of medicine includes the promotion of medicine. There must be a "treatment". A treatment that promotes medical procedures and medicinal drugs. A treatment that usually restrains the immune system so that the disease becomes more difficult, if not impossible, to defeat.

The American Cancer Society (ACS) sits proudly in its plush offices. Its chief officer receives hundreds of thousands of dollars in salary. Thanks to a brainwashed public, there is no end to the funding the society receives.

Millions and millions of dollars pour into their coffers. The Jimmy Fund is a great tool of the cancer people. "If you love the children you will donate generously", and the American people being generous, donate billions to the cancer societies. Most of the money goes for salaries and operating expenses. The American Cancer Society may not do too well at finding a cure for cancer; but they are very generous with their payment to their officers and directors. All said and done, an amount equal to not much more than 10% of their gross is used for research. Research to find a cure that has eluded them for 100 years is the least of their problems. Their main interest is funding. There is no limit to the amount of funding they will accept in their search for a "cure". Their main sales pitch is, "The cure is on the horizon." And the cure will always be on the horizon for the American Cancer Society, unless the American people wake up and look at the monster that hovers over them.

The American Cancer Society has close connections to the mammography industry. Five radiologists have served as ACS presidents, and the ACS promotes the interests of the major manufacturers of mammogram machines and films, including Siemens, DuPont, General Electric, Eastman Kodak, and Piker. The mammography industry also conducts research for the ACS and its grantees, serves on advisory boards, and donates considerable funds. DuPont is a substantial backer of the ACS Breast Health Awareness Program. It sponsors television shows and other media productions touting mammography. It produces advertising, promotional, and information literature for hospitals, clinics, medical organizations, and doctors. It produces educational films; and, of course, it lobbies Congress for legislation promoting the availability of mammography services. Since mammography screening is a profit-driven technology, the ACS has been and remains strongly linked with the mammography industry.

The "irony" of mammograms is that breast tissue is bombarded with a type of radiation that, with sufficient exposure, will cause cancer. Women over forty are urged to get at least two mammograms a year (two exposures of radiation a year). With sufficient exposure, cancer finally appears and the doctors proudly boast to have "caught it in the early stages." If there had been no mammograms performed, then likely breast cancer would not have occurred. Instead the hapless victims are relieved it was discovered "in the early stages" and happily accept chemo over mutilation as their only early choice for survival. They never associate those semi-annual radiation treatments with the generation of their breast cancers.

The search for a cancer cure has proven to be one of the most lucrative markets in our society. It must be said that the American Cancer Society has not cornered the cancer cure market. Dana-Farber Institute is right there in the running. They are not slouches, with David Nathan, President Emeritus, taking home a cool million in salary. The Cancer Research Institute lags slightly behind with Executive Director Jill O'Donnell-Torme with a mere $335,000.

There are others who have cut themselves in for a piece of the action. Some lesser known names as Multiple Myeloma Research Foundation with executive director Scott Santarella with only $200,000.

Breast cancer has become big business simply because they haven't found the cause or the cure. Like other medical research societies, not finding the cause or cure keeps these lucrative ventures alive and well. Finding the cause and cure of a disease or disorder, even though that has never happened, would be the end of that particular program.

Radiation from routine mammography poses significant risks of initiating and promoting benign tumors in the patient receiving the X-rays. They are creating their own diseases. Once the patient develops 2 or 3 benign tumors, the doctor may then biopsy of one of the tumors, causing that particular tumor to become malignant. This may then be followed by chemotherapy, which suppresses the immune system and which leads to cancer of the entire bloodstream. This is often followed by more drugs and often leads to a horrible death. Convention assures us that radiation exposure from mammography is trivial. That is, according to "medical studies and statistics". It is not true according to anyone who has the ability to see and possesses the ability to believe what he sees. An interesting note, not to my surprise, Myra Biblowit, President of The Breast Cancer Research Foundation receives an annual salary of $500,000!

Patients who do not survive the outrageous cancer treatments being touted by the cancer industry today, are too many to count; and the medical authorities do not want to count. They do not want to know. The medical authorities need only to wait for that one exception who happens to survive the medical "treatments" being perpetrated on cancer patients, that one exception who happened to survive biopsy, surgery, chemotherapy and/or radiation and who actually appears to be a survivor of the disease. That particular patient is then paraded before the American public by such outlets as CNN Television. One exceptional example is that of Lance Armstrong. Although he is one in a bazillion, his remarkable story offers blind acceptance in modern medicine and cancer victims everywhere believe they can be "cured" just like him.

The public is made aware of an imaginary miracle of modern medicine and is led to believe that cancer-cure is the rule; but the fact is, cancer-cure is not the rule. The immune system has the ability to deal successfully with the disease; but it has a nearly impossible job when it has to deal with the disease as well as the "treatments" at the same time! The American people are being taken for a ride, not only by the medical industry, but also by the media over which the medical industry exerts great control.

Only children and the very strong, can survive the outrageous, self-serving practices of an industry gone wild. An industry that has learned the value of brainwashing. Only a brainwashed person can believe that 100 years of cancer research without a cure is an excellent record. Only a brainwashed person can believe that 100 years of research without a cure deserves to be rewarded with billions of dollars in funding. A report issued by the American Cancer Society a few years ago found a staggering 150 Americans per hour were diagnosed with cancer. They also claimed that cancer cures are becoming more frequent. That is exactly correct. The reason so many Americans are being diagnosed with cancer is that so many Americans are taking medicine. The reason cures are more frequent is that more people, after being diagnosed with cancer, are turning away from mainstream medicine. More people are turning away from radiation, mammography and especially chemotherapy —the great depressor of the immune system and the great killer!

The ACS recently held a fund balance of over $400 million with about $69 million worth of holdings in real estate, office buildings, and equipment. How this helps them to cure cancer remains a well-hidden secret. How they could spend billions of dollars without finding a cure is mind boggling; but the fact is that a cure was found. It was found and was so unacceptable to the authorities that it was shunned like the plague.

The fact is that cancer is very much preventable and very much curable. There are those in the industry who are aware of this fact but still remain silent. The great breakthrough came in the 1970's. It was found patients receiving large amounts of immunosuppressive drugs in order to receive organ transplants, developed Kaposi's Sarcoma, a skin cancer. The doctors halted the drugs while contemplating what caused the cancer and what treatment they might employ. The doctors, after stopping the drug treatment and while pondering their next step, found that the cancerous tumors either diminished in size or disappeared completely. —AIDS, The Mystery and the Solution by Alan Cantwell, Jr. M.D.

This was shocking. The possibility that at least one form of cancer was caused by medicinal drugs would be somewhat upsetting to the drug industry, to say the least. To find that a cure for anything, let alone cancer, could be achieved by the discontinuance of medicine was something that had to be carefully studied. The thought that other forms of cancer or other diseases could be caused by medicine was unacceptable to an industry bent on the promotion and sales of drugs. What happened then is unknown, but a real breakthrough had occurred and was then quietly put to sleep. The possibility that cancer could be caused by medicinal drugs and cured by the withdrawal of those drugs was not to be accepted by medical authorities. That cancer was caused by drugs would be devastating to the pharmaceutical industry. The best thing to do was to completely ignore these findings and that is apparently just what they did. The authorities decided to treat these findings as if they had never taken place. They did exactly that and to date they never looked back. Today, drugs are used in the treatment of cancer and Americans are dying by the thousands.

Billions of dollars pour into medical research foundations, most of which goes into everything but research. All of it is an unnecessary waste. Even the funds that actually do go into research are a complete waste of the public's money. The medical paraphernalia, the drugs, the buildings, the offices, the entire panorama, strictly show business! A gigantic scam! The fact is that cancer is curable by the immune system, a 60 trillion cellular universe all by itself. It is estimated that the averaged sized adult is composed of 60 trillion cells working in concert for its own good. A universe of 60 trillion cells that have the ability to prevent or cure any disease under the sun. 60 trillion cells, the understanding of which the medical experts haven't even come close to scratching the surface. For anyone and for any reason, to insert a droplet of poison into this star-sent universe, to tamper with it in any way so as to "improve on its workings" is nothing less than a crime against the patient and a crime against nature. When done by force or by government mandate or for the purpose of financial gain, it becomes a crime against humanity.

SCHERING-PLOUGH

One of our great pharmaceutical companies!

Are these companies our benefactors, or are we dealing with criminal organizations? The answer remains to be seen. The question remains: "Can we allow an organization, such as Schering-Plough, Eli Lilly and others to force their products on us, our children or even our household pets?" There is no question that forced medicine is now in the planning stages and quickly approaching, thanks to ObamaCare Socialized Medicine. Our children and we have become sitting ducks for an industry that has become crazed with profits and power!

Schering-Plough to admit guilt, pay $435M fine in fraud probe.

Drugmaker's latest scandal centers on cancer medicine.

Wednesday, August 30, 2006

BY George E. Jordan

Star-Ledger (Newark NJ) Staff

"Schering-Plough yesterday said it would plead guilty to criminal conspiracy and pay a $435,000 fine to settle a federal investigation into fraud, kickbacks and illegal sales and marketing tactics. The payout brings to $1 billion the criminal and civil penalties paid by the Kenilworth-based drug maker in recent years to settle allegations of illegal business practices under former Chief Executive Richard Kogan."

Schering-Plough gave $295,000 to federal candidates in the 2006 election. In that year the company spent $1,800,000 through its political action committee.

Fred Hassan, CEO gets $1,650,000 annual salary. Other executives get over $500,000. Schering-Plough Corporation merged with Merck & Co. on November 4th, 2009. Merck; a company that has known even more notoriety than Schering-Plough was an interesting choice! This is a marriage that bears watching, and a marriage, certainly not one made in heaven.

Eli Lilly settles Zyprexa lawsuit for $1.42 billion

Associated Press Thurs., Jan. 15, 2009

(Excerpts)

"INDIANAPOLIS – Eli Lilly & Co. said Thursday it pleaded guilty to a charge that it illegally marketed the anti-psychotic drug Zyprexa for an unapproved use,

and will pay $1.42 billion to settle civil suits and end the criminal investigation.

"The Indianapolis-based company said it will pay $800 million to settle civil suits, including $438 million to the federal government and $362 million to states. It will pay $615 million to resolve the criminal probe, and plead guilty to a misdeameanor violation of the Food, Drug and Cosmetic Act for promoting Zyprexa as a dementia treatment."

"Earlier the same month, Lilly agreed to pay $62 million to 32 states and the District of Columbia to resolve accusations it marketed Zyprexa for pediatric care, for use in high doses and for dementia."

Johnson & Johnson Accused of Drug Kickbacks
New York Times

By NATASHA SINGER

Published: January 15, 2010

(Excerpt)

"Johnson & Johnson paid kickbacks to the nation's largest nursing home pharmacy to increase the number of elderly patients taking the antipsychotic Risperdal and several other medications, accorcding to a complaint filed Friday by the office of the United States attorney in Boston.

"The payments violated the federal anti-kickback statute and led Omnicare, a pharmacy company specializing in dispensing drugs to nursing home residents, to submit false claims to Medicaid the complaint charged.

"The government's civil complaint joins a whistle-blower suit against Johnson & Johnson brought by two former employees of Omnicare, which has headquarters in Covington, Ky.

"The complaint charges that Omnicare's pharmacists engaged in intensive efforts to persuade physicians to prescribe the drugs from 1999 to 2004, a period in which the pharmacy's annual purchase of Johnson & Johnson medications nearly tripled to more than $280 million, from about $100 million. During the same period, the pharmacy's annual purchase of Risperdal rose to more than $100 million, according to the complaint filed in United States District Court in Massachusetts."

Cancers, even advanced cancers, can sometimes undergo what is called 'spontaneous regression' - i.e., they can simply disappear without trace. Spontaneous regression is much more common than the medical industry would have us believe. It is the immune system doing its work. Yet, this wonderful cure for a dread disease can be hampered by an assault on the immune system; and that is exactly what happens when the patient is drugged. The medical authorities have no interest in hearing about a cure that is achieved without medicine, no interest in studying such a cure, and complete refusal to let it interfere with the status quo even though they themselves have not found a cure for over 100 years of research.

6. Vaccinations

To inject a vile morbid substance into the body of an infant, all in the name of profits, is one of the greatest possible crimes against children, society and humanity that I can contemplate. Apart from increased susceptibility to the disease itself, immune dysfunctions, multiple sclerosis, metabolic disease, gastrointestinal disease, organ failure, allergic enteropathy (intestinal disease), and severe intestinal damage, neurological disorders, diabetes, dozens of other diseases and sometimes death result from these directly injected poisons into the human body.

The actual frequency of negative results cannot be known because doctors are not given any real incentive to report adverse effects. They are also told that they must never let their patients (or parents) think that the risks could outweigh the benefits. Doctors must create their own statistics, and they do. Since there are no benefits, the risks certainly do outweigh the benefits.

An honest study would show that unvaccinated children are noticeably stronger, healthier, more alert, more aware, and happier than those vaccinated. They learn faster and are ahead of their peers at school. Hundreds of babies and young children die and/or are permanently brain-damaged each year here in the United States following "routine" vaccinations! Proof that tampering with the immune system can cause devastating disease and death. Half a million children in this country alone suffer from autism which thousands of parents attribute to vaccinations.

"But thousands of children cared for by Homefirst Health Services in metropolitan Chicago have at least two things in common with thousands of Amish children in rural Lancaster: They have never been vaccinated. And they don't have autism. "We have a fairly large practice. We have about 30,000 or 35,000 children that we've taken care of over the years, and I don't think we have a single case of autism in children delivered by us who never received vaccines," said Dr. Mayer Eisenstein, Homefirst's medical director who founded the practice in 1973.

The vaccine industry remains comatose. They will not give in —they will win no matter what. They have the secret weapon. The most important asset belongs to them. Do they have something that will benefit society? The answer is "No!" —They have very little to benefit anyone; but they can win! They will pedal their products around the entire planet, they will do it by force if necessary; and what is their secret weapon against those who will not be duped? Against those who refuse to be brought into the fold? Against those who refuse to be poisoned? Their secret weapon is Deep Pockets and world leaders and elected officials who are willing to sell out their constituents.

Chemical diseases injected into the human body are not exactly what nature had in mind for the child, or even for the adult. Nature's plan is to bring on diseases to the child in a natural way. By so doing, the child obtains lifetime immunity, not only to the childhood diseases but especially asthma and allergies, and to strains of these diseases that encompass many, if not all other diseases.

Once the baby's immune system has been assaulted by continuous piercing, especially for the purpose of injecting morbid matter into the tiny body, that child will have damaged and compromised health for life. The immune system can heal itself. The immune system can recover from nearly any trauma; but it seems that it does not recover completely from the violent act of vaccination. The immune system appears to be forever compromised by vaccination. There is no question whatsoever in my own mind that much of disease in society today originates with childhood vaccinations.

Could vaccines be weakening the immune system of our populations and causing asthma and allergies at unprecedented levels? I believe the answer to be "Yes!" Amazingly, the medical profession ignores the incriminating evidence against vaccines, and continues to inflict more unnecessary harm on society at large, not the least of which is our nation's infants! Every time I hear of the tragic death of an infant, I have to suspect a vaccine was at work, even though I have never known of an autopsy, a doctor, or a doctor's assistant to make any such admission.

The vaccination hoax is the most outrageous superstition modern medicine has managed to impose, but, also the most profitable. There is not a shred of evidence that vaccination has any value. Except of course, medical "statistics".

There is no doubt that autism and other diseases are caused by the brain's reaction to the morbid matter that makes its way into the bloodstream.

The promoters of vaccines will do nothing about this until the lawsuits outweigh the profits, which will never happen while our elected officials prevent these lawsuits. The National Vaccine Injury Compensation Program (VICP) is a federal program that was passed by US Congress to compensate families for injuries and death as a direct result of vaccinations. Vaccines are enormously profitable for drug companies and recent legislation in the US has exempted lawsuits against pharmaceutical firms in the event of adverse reactions to vaccines, which are very common. Vaccine-makers are shielded so they would not go bankrupt as a result of being sued for vaccine-injuries. The National Vaccine Injury Compensation Program has already passed the billion-dollar mark in claims for vaccine-caused injuries and deaths; and with forced vaccinations, the industry will reap gigantic profits while the American People will pay, not only physically but also financially, for the devastation caused by these products.

Immunization (the act of injecting vaccines) depresses and disables brain and immune function. Honest, unbiased scientific investigation has shown vaccinations to be a causative factor in many illnesses including:

Sudden Infant Death Syndrome also known as SIDS or crib or cot death, developmental disorders, Autism, seizures, mental retardation, hyperactivity, Dyslexia and many others. A rise in peanut allergies and other severe allergic reactions in young people, and even older people, both acute and chronic, is associated with a rise in childhood vaccinations. This could be easily proven or disproved if the vaccine industry and/or their colleagues were willing to examine this possibility. They're not willing. They don't want to know. They are well protected by our elected officials, the media, our courts, and even a brainwashed public.

Every vile substance injected into the human body has its own, often disastrous, effects. Dr. Gherardi emphasizes that once aluminum is injected into the muscle, the immune activation persists for years. In addition, we must consider the effect of the aluminum that travels to the brain itself. Numerous studies have shown harmful effects when aluminum accumulates in the brain.

A growing amount of evidence points to high brain aluminum levels as a major contributor to Alzheimer's disease and possibly Parkinson's disease and ALS (Lou Gehrig's disease).

This may also explain the tenfold increase in Alzheimer's disease in those receiving the flu vaccine five years in a row. (Dr. Hugh Fudenberg, in press, Journal of Clinical Investigation).

Drug makers are especially afraid of lawsuits stemming from vaccines that, unlike drugs, are given to healthy people, making any harm they cause an even bigger legal risk. What is not being addressed besides all of the filthy ingredients of vaccines, is the fact that just the plain violation of the body, especially that of an infant, is enough to activate an immune response.

----- Original Message -----

From: Daniel H Duffy Sr.

To: drsfosterdc@aol.com

Sent: Saturday, February 09, 2002 7:49 AM

Subject: VACCINE OPINION

"I am in receipt of a letter concerning public action on vaccines. "The letter points out the manner in which unelected officials in government beauroacracies begin to rob the citizen of his fundamental rights and freedoms. It should be immediately recognized as such. "Those people attempting to force ANY type of compulsory or mandatory medical technique of ANY type other than quarantine for a short period of time [a necessity unlikely ever to occur] i.e., CDC, NIH, etc should be recognized as criminals and treated as such. They are violating the constitutionally guaranteed rights of citizens and are in violation of the principles laid down at Nuremberg over fifty years ago.

"We must stop indulging in polite conversations with these people, they are NOT scientists, they are on the public dole and they are robbing us of our tax monies to support their nefarious roles in government, to wit, to support organized medicine and the pharmaceutical interests.

"There is no such thing as a safe vaccine. The fact that this is so easily established from the historical

record magnifies the terrible force with which we must reckon.

"No vaccine ever prevented, ameliorated or cured any disease as the record, when properly interpreted or re-interpreted proves.

"Every vaccine is a form of Russian Roulette and vaccination must be placed in the closet of medical quackery along with the rest of the drug driven nonsense of the 20th century.

"Until reasonable men come to this conclusion the vaccine makers and drug makers will continue to hold sway.

"They are NOT scientists, they are QUACKS. The real problem is that when someone, such as I, stands up and identifies them as such, I [WE] are considered the quacks. That exemplifies how far down the road we are and how difficult it is going to be finally extricate them.

"You must ask yourself, wherein lies the quackery of the ESTABLISHMENT today? Keeping in mind that EVERY age has its own peculiar form of ESTABLISHMENT quackery and that this age is NO exception to THAT rule.

"I have studied the vaccine situation since first vaccinated at my induction into the military in 1947. I spent the next 21 years avoiding my next vaccination and I very carefully invesigated the effects of vaccination. I can tell you that it is the worst horror story imaginable and no one, not even the antivaccinationists have the slightest clue as to exactly how horrible that story is."

Daniel H Duffy Sr DC

Small town family doctor, 30 years.

Retired Air Force Officer 21 years.

****

"There is a great deal of evidence to prove that immunization of children does more harm than good. There is no evidence that any influenza vaccine thus far developed is effective in preventing or mitigating any attack of influenza. The producers of these vaccines know that they are worthless, but they go on selling them, anyway." —Dr. J. Anthony Morris (formerly Chief Vaccine Control Officer at the FDA).

The drug industry is not satisfied with the status quo. They have won. They have complete control of our Congress as far as their industry is concerned. They have become the law of the land, and are stopping nowhere and at nothing. They have a long reach. Lobbyists have reached Iraq. They may not be referred to as lobbyists, but Iraq is now poised to become the next victim. The World Health Organization and UNICEF are overseeing the work of 8,000 volunteers who aim to give up to 3.9 million children the MMR vaccine. A completely worthless product like all other vaccines but with the ability to cause sickness, disease, death and to subject thousands of Iraqi children to the disease of autism. The drug promoters continue to search for new markets. When they don't find one, they make one.

CHINESE POLICE ARREST VACCINATION PROTESTERS!

National Vaccine Information Center Newsletter

"Chinese police hauled off a small group of people on Thursday who had arrived in Beijing's Tiananmen

Square to protest what they say are bad vaccines which have crippled their children, one of the demonstrators said. They say that their children were vaccinated against Japanese encephalitis B in 2003 in the southern province of Guangdong, and that the vaccine has paralyzed their sons and daughters. China's Health Ministry told Reuters last month that they had found no problem with the vaccines."—Reuters, Beijing, Aug. 17, 2006

Lobbyists are not confined to the Halls of Congress

Tom Blackwell

National Post

Tuesday, December 03, 2002

(Excerpt)

"Numerous Canadians who got flu shots last year had negative reactions ranging from swelling of the brain to anaphylactic shock and total paralysis, says an exhaustive new Health Canada report.

"Others suffered convulsions, vomiting and chest pains, the department revealed in one of the most extensive studies ever conducted in Canada into the side effects of vaccination."

I have traced numerous diseases to vaccination. Autism and Down's syndrome among many others. The list is long. A board of statisticians, with no interest in the sales, manufacture or promotion of these vile products, would find that scores of diseases for which there is no apparent cause can be traced to vaccinations. Diseases ranging from tumors, to severe allergic reactions both acute and chronic, Alzheimer's among many others. Vaccines are definitely weakening the immune system of our populations and causing asthma and allergies at unprecedented levels. I have found that children who were vaccinated, do not enjoy the health of those unvaccinated such as the Amish, and certain other religious groups like the Christian Scientists.

According to recent news items, thousands of American children have acquired autism. My own findings are that autism exists only where vaccination exists. It is unheard of among the Amish in Pennsylvania who do not vaccinate. Still, the medical industry has been able to provide "proof" enough to satisfy a court of law, that autism is never due to vaccination.

We have not only lost the loyalty of our elected officials, the media, the doctors, but even the courts have been brought into the fold. We have nowhere to turn but to the Internet, word of mouth, and the free press. Who will betray us next? Word of mouth may be ours to keep; but the free press and the Internet still remain a thorn in the side of the medical authorities. I'm sure these freedoms are being scrutinized by the medical industry as we speak. These are the last two barriers to FORCED MEDICINE! The last two barriers that keep us from that slippery slope and that road of no return.

Just recently, Dr. Max Wiznitzer, a key vaccine proponent admitted on a Friday night US TV program "Larry King Live" that the rate of Autism in Northeastern Ohio, the largest Amish community in the USA with low rates of vaccination, was 1 in 10,000. He should know, he said: *"I'm their neurologist."* The rate among vaccinated children is about 1 in 150 and climbing.

THE US MEDICAL INDUSTRY AGAIN REACHES OUT!

MMR docs' links with drugs firms

Feb 29, 2004

By Fionnuala Burke, Sunday Mercury

"Four leading doctors who deemed the controversial MMR vaccine safe have links to the drug giants who make or supply the jab.

"Professor James Chipman from Birmingham University, a member of the Committee on Safety of Medicines, received research funding from GlaxoSmithKline, suppliers of the MMR vaccine Priorix.

"Consultant cardiologist Dr Colin Forfar from John Radcliffe Hospital in Oxford, a shareholder in GlaxoSmithKline, is also a member of the influential committee.

"Professor Terence Stephenson, from the Queen's Medical Centre in Nottingham, sits on the same committee but his travel expenses are paid by the same drug giant.

"Professor Michael Langman from Birmingham University is the Chairman of the Joint Committee on Vaccination and Immunization. His team received research support from Merck Sharp and Dohme, which manufactures MMR vaccine.

"Now Jonathan Harris, West Midlands campaigner for vaccination awareness group JABS (Justice Awareness and Basic Support) is calling for the GMC to investigate the work of the medics. Only two of Mr. Harris's six children had the MMR vaccine and both of them are autistic. These experts are advising the Government about the safety of the MMR vaccine at the same time as receiving payments or holding shares in the companies selling the jab." —©2004 Independent Newspapers (UK) Limited".

Ten Reasons to Just Say "No!" to Vaccinations

Idaho Observer

Vaccinations are toxins by definition.

Vaccinations are aggressively promoted by those who have a financial stake in their consumption.

Vaccinations are promoted using fear, intimidation, and coercion.

Vaccinations are big business.

Vaccine manufacturers are liability-proof for their products.

Vaccinations are not only forced upon us, but those who deny us the exercise of our free will refuse to take responsibility for the consequences of their actions.

Evidence suggests that vaccinations damage the immune system, the nervous system and the spirit-mind-body connection.

Compulsory vaccinations ignore biochemical and psycho-spiritual individuality.

Vaccinations are misrepresented by government agencies as a public health issue, which they are not.

Vaccinations are heavily subsidized, heavily propagandized and can be seen as a wake-up call for us to see how we allow ourselves to be programmed by huge vested interests.

Christian Scientists, by abstaining from vaccinations and many other medical procedures, enjoy such excellent health, when they do acquire an ailment; they are able to recover at their Sanatoriums or Christian Science Benevolent Centers. These facilities are on a par with our mainstream hospitals, fully paid by many of the large insurance companies. The great insurance companies find it extremely profitable to sell health insurance to Christian Scientists since these people enjoy such excellent health. Christian Scientists credit much of their Health Care success to prayer; but I suggest they get fewer diseases and recover more rapidly from their ailments because of their rejection of vaccinations and other medicines. Honest investigation would find no evidence whatsoever that any vaccine ever prevented or helped to prevent any disease or disorder. The only proof that exists is the word of the government agencies, fabricated medical statistics, and the refusal of members of Congress to betray their lobbyist benefactors.

The 1993 Comprehensive Childhood Immunization Act, signed by President Clinton, gave the Department of Health and Human Services (HHS) $400 million to set up state vaccine registries. These tag and track children so they can be compelled to receive vaccinations.

The success of the Polio Vaccine is the great credential of the medical industry. It is paraded before us over and over by the media and other forms of advertising. The fact is that when the truth is known, this vaccine and all others may be toppled into the dust!

"Of course Polio was here before the Polio vaccine; but the Polio death rate was decreasing on its own before the vaccine was introduced, and cases of Polio increased after mass inoculations. The United States Centers for Disease Control once admitted that the vaccine has become the dominant cause of Polio in the US with 87% of cases between 1973 and 1983 caused by the vaccine. More recently, in 1980-1989 according to CDC figures, every case of Polio in the US was caused by the vaccine." http://www.whale.to/vaccines/polio.html

"In 1956, with the infamous Francis Field Trials, it was discovered that large numbers of children contracted Polio after receiving the vaccine. Instead of removing the vaccine from the market, they decided to exclude from the statistics all cases of Polio that occurred within 30 days after vaccination on the pretext that such cases were "pre-existing." www.thinktwice.com

"Use of the Salk vaccine will increase the possibility that your child will contact the disease. It appears that the most effective way to protect your child from Polio is to make sure that he does not get the vaccine." Dr. Robert Mendelsohn (1984).

Where Polio vaccination programs have been instituted worldwide, reported polio infections show a 700% increase as a result of compulsory vaccination. In 1958, mass vaccination triggered a disastrous increase in Polio, the highest being 700% in Ottawa, Canada. The highest incidence in the USA occurred in those states that had been induced to adopt compulsory

Polio shots. Statistics on Polio were manipulated. New diagnostic guidelines were issued by the CDC: if you object to Polio vaccination, and you get Polio —it is usually called "Polio." If you have been vaccinated and you get "Polio", it is called Meningitis. —http://www. nccn.net/~wwithin/polio2.htm

"The Salk vaccine has been directly responsible for the major increase in Leukemia in this country."— Dr. Klenner, M.D.

"Within a few years of the polio vaccine we started seeing some strange phenomena. For instance, the year before the first 300,000 doses were given in the United States, childhood Leukemia had never struck a child under the age of two. One year after the first onslaught they had the first cases of children under the age of two that died of leukemia. Dr. Herbert Radnor observed that in a small area of this little town, an area where no cases of Leukemia had been expected or at the most one in 4 years according to previous statistics, they suddenly had a rash like an epidemic within a few blocks."— Dr. Snead

Dr. Benjamin Sandler observed that children consume greater amounts of ice cream, soda pop, and artificially sweetened products. In 1949, before the polio season began, he warned the residents of North Carolina, through newspapers and radio, to decrease their consumption of these products. During that summer North Carolinians reduced their intake of sugar by 90% and polio decreased in that state in 1949 by the same amount. (One manufacturer shipped one million less gallons of ice cream during the first week alone following the publication of Dr. Sandler's anti-polio diet.

Coca Cola sales were down as well. But the powerful Rockefeller Milk Trust, which sold frozen products to North Carolinians, combined forces with the Coca Cola power merchants and convinced people that Sandler's findings were a myth and the polio figures a fluke. By the summer of 1950 sales were back to ordinary levels and polio cases returned to "normal" during that year.)

Not only did the polio vaccine have nothing to do with the decline of polio, evidence shows that vaccinations for this and other diseases —notably diphtheria and smallpox were responsible for its increase. The decline of cases not caused by vaccination began to disappear in the West with improvements in hygiene and sanitation and most of the decline occurred well before the widespread use of polio vaccination.

There is no question that studies and tests by the medical industry can produce whatever results they desire. Not only are vaccines worthless in preventing disease they are counterproductive because they injure the immune system permitting cancer, autoimmune diseases and SIDS, and cause much disability and death.

The vaccine business is about to explode. Watch out for public health officials and pharmaceutical industry lobbyists, who will descend on state legislatures and push for mandatory vaccination laws. Americans may be told it is their patriotic duty to take vaccinations whether they want to or not, in order to finance the development and stockpiling of flu vaccine for a flu pandemic that may or may not occur. And when people get hurt by mandated flu vaccination, they will be left to fend for themselves just like most victims of mandated childhood vaccines are left to fend for themselves. The majority of child vaccine victims are turned away from the federal Vaccine Injury Compensation Program created in 1986 by Congress.

The CDC (Centers for Disease Control) has drafted a model law which will require forced vaccinations of all Americans, imprisonment and quarantine of those who refuse to submit to vaccination, seizure of property and other drastic measures. Vaccination is one of the most controversial aspects of medicine. While the official position of the medical establishment is that vaccination is a foundation of public health policy, thousands of doctors and hundreds of millions of people worldwide consider it to be a leading cause of disease, neurological damage, learning disabilities and death and to be ineffective in conferring immunity.

Crib Death was so infrequent in the pre-vaccination era that it was not even mentioned in the statistics, but it started to climb in the 1950s with the spread of mass vaccination against diseases of childhood. According to my own findings, this syndrome is almost always connected to vaccinations. But the medical establishment assures us that SIDS (Sudden Infant Death Syndrome) is unrelated to vaccinations. How do they know? They don't really want to know. All they need is an answer to satisfy the skeptics. A satisfactory alibi so they can continue down their chosen path. The answer is simple. They have "statistics". No matter how obvious it is that the incidence of SIDS following childhood vaccines is great, the medical authorities, along with their partners in Congress, the media, the courts, and a brainwashed public, have exact and precise statistics. Statistics that, even though they have no basis in fact, have become the law of the land. They need only be spoken by the authorities to become validated. To question these statistics has been called un-American. Failure to believe medical statistics and follow their lead has resulted in criminal indictment and even imprisonment. Americans no longer have the right to question or disagree with medical authority! If this has a familiar ring to it, remember Nazi Germany!

Recently there has been quite an "epidemic" of the so-called "shaken baby syndrome". Parents, usually the fathers or other caregivers such as nannies, have increasingly been accused of shaking a baby to the point of causing permanent brain damage and death. Why? Is there an unprecedented increase in the number of people who commit infanticide or have an ambition to seriously hurt babies? Or is there something more sinister at play? Japan changed the start time for vaccinating from three months to two years and straight away their SIDS rate plummeted:

"Delay of DPT immunization until 2 years of age in Japan has resulted in a dramatic decline in adverse side effects. In the period of 1970-1974, when DPT vaccination was begun at 3 to 5 months of age, the Japanese national compensation system paid out claims for 57 permanent severe damage vaccine cases, and 37 deaths. During the ensuing six-year period 1975-1980, when DPT injections were delayed to 24 months of age, severe reactions from the vaccine were reduced to a total of eight with three deaths. This represents an 85 to 90 percent reduction in severe cases of damage and death." —Raymond Obomsawin, M.D.

In every single case of SIDS that I have come across, the symptoms appeared shortly after the baby's vaccinations. We have witnessed a steady rise in the incidence of SIDS, closely following the growth in childhood vaccinations.

My suspicion, which is shared by others, is that the nearly 10,000 SIDS deaths that occur in the United States each year are related to one or more of the vaccines that are routinely given children.

7. Epilogue

Drugs are not the cure; they are the cause of disease. The use of drugs and vaccinations in the treatment and prevention of disease should be abolished. It does not work, it never did and never will, except according to the "studies" and "statistics" created by those in the business of promoting these products. When someone dies from this stuff called "medicine", that happens every minute of every day, doctors are well versed in how to cover up. The death certificate might read "heart failure" or some pre-existing condition. When someone dies from a vaccine or even the flu shot, which happens more often than you think, once again the death certificate might read "heart failure" or whatever is the whim of the doctor. The drug companies manage to keep a somewhat clean slate. I find that the Number One cause of sickness, disease, premature death, birth defects and even crime in our society is medicinal drugs. What part do medicinal drugs play in this world of turmoil? What does the assault and pollution of the bloodstream by medicinal drugs have to do with the evil perpetrated by so many leaders and others around the world?

That remains to be seen. I have found from my own observations that the unexplainable mass murders that take place in our society today are not caused by those who failed to take their medicine, but by those who did take it. Children who commit suicide and children who kill are not children who failed to take their Prozac. They are children who did take it. Nothing causes more depression than anti-depressants! Mothers who drown their children for no apparent reason did not fail to take their medicine, as the authorities would have us believe. They are those who did take it. The Jeffrey Dahmers of the world are almost always those who took their medicine, or the products of mothers who took theirs. We can stop the high rate of crime, the diseases for which no cure can be found, even the budget deficit, by stopping the use of drugs or that poison called "medicine".

It may prove to be the Number One cause of our Nation's earth-shattering problems and may even be a major cause of world leaders who prefer violence to peace. As if that were not enough, I suggest in time, what we have come to know as "medicine" will prove to be the Number One cause of the pollution of the earth's water supply.

I have found that when the vilest substances are in our bloodstream, the closer we come to cancer and premature death. The more vile the substances we ingest into our systems the more we induce disease and illness. The immune system has the ability to protect us from disease, and to defeat disease; but it must be unpolluted and it must be allowed and encouraged to do its pre-ordained work.

Because of the power of brainwashing and Deep Pockets, the drug industry may continue to prosper; but those of us who have managed to escape their grasp must demand and fight if necessary, for the right to reject medical treatment especially when we have found something that works better. We must demand the right to employ natural healing or natural immunity when we believe it is superior to that manufactured in a pharmaceutical laboratory.

Nearly every disease in our society can be, and more than often has been, caused by pharmaceutical drugs. We have been overwhelmed by FDA "studies" and "statistics". We have been brainwashed, browbeaten, intimidated and forced by law, at times with police power, to submit to the demands of the creators of these statistics as well as to their morbid and vile products.

The US Government has not been able to convince the world to employ the great system of democracy. Our elected officials have failed to convince the people of the world that peace and prosperity are better than violence and despair; but our Leaders, in league with the Medical Industry have spent trillions of dollars and have succeeded in convincing just about everyone on the planet that the intake of poison can be beneficial to the human body. Once again the question, "Who are our representatives serving; the American People or the Medical Industry?"

I suggest that a study by statisticians, who have no interest in the status quo of American Medicine, who have no interest in the outcome of the study, who have no personal agenda and no fear of repercussions from the powers that be, could easily prove that the use of vaccinations and drugs in the prevention and treatment of disease is the greatest fraud ever perpetrated on the human race.

Letters

Letter from Ray Gallup to Congressman Burton and read at the December 10, 2002 hearing:

"I was set to go with Albert Enayati tomorrow for the Government reform hearings but could not make it. Our family is in living hell with our 17 year-old son Eric who is 6 feet tall, 150 pounds. He attacked Helen, Julie, my daughter (14) and myself. He head butted Julie and bit my wife on the head. Eric bit one of my fingers. It is not the first time and is getting worse. We have no help and I'm afraid for the safety of our family and my son.

"He is a victim of Merck...with the MMR vaccine...having elevated measles antibody titers.

"Eric was like he was 6'-5" and 300 pounds on Sunday when he had his tantrum. I held him down but he tried to bite me and kick and scratch me. I was so exhausted I could not breathe and thought I would have a heart attack. When we closed the doors to lock ourselves in from Eric, Eric kicked on the door...breaking some of the wood.

"I do not know what to do anymore short of calling the police...we are at our wits end.

"This is our lot in life for trusting the medical profession that vaccines are safe. We are paying a bitter price for that trust. It is hard to have any holiday feelings

when we see what has happened to our son...and our family.

"Again, I am sorry I could not attend but we are under siege".

Ray Gallup

****

H E Sri A P J Abdul Kalam Azad,

Hon'ble President of India,

Rashtrapati Bhawan,

New Delhi.

Dt: 29.08.2006

Most Respected Sir,

"We vaccine damage victims and the parents of vaccine-damaged children have been raising our voices against the vile practice of vaccines for quite a long time now. We know that nobody is really interested in our problems, created by Government-sponsored mass vaccine programs indulged in without apprising us of the dangers involved. But we continue regardless not for our sake, our lives have already changed forever for the worst, but for the children who are choosing this country to evolve in their spiritual quest.

"Little do those children know that India is no longer the country it once was. Today the love for mankind the country possessed, the spiritual nature of its people and its great system of education aiming at generating and advancing humane knowledge has been lost. In the name of science we have changed. Science is

supposed to be a search for the truth but today the truth is being suppressed in the name of science.

"Where will our movement end? As the enclosed report states, the Chinese Government is now arresting vaccine protestors. We too may be arrested and put behind bars. We are being termed a 'hazard to public health'. What health, Sir? We no longer see health around us, but only death and disease. Yet we talk of public health. We spend billions so that the medical industry prospers and thrives. Nobody thinks of the patients anymore and what they are being forced to go through, health wise and finance wise, at the hands of this evil industry.

"We are at fault for pointing out that vaccines are a bundle of extremely toxic, carcinogenic and contaminated elements that are being forcibly pushed into young defenseless children who cannot protest, whose parents are not aware of the dangers, whose sacrifice of life, and its opportunities go towards filling the coffers of the medical industry which prefers to bow down to the dictate of agencies who have long since lost their sanctity and credibility in the eyes of the general population all over the world.

"What sort of an age do we live in, Sir? We are forced to part with both our health and life's income to promote an industry that peddles death and disease in return. Is this what our freedom fighters laid down their lives for? Is this what Gandhiji gave his life for? Is this the expression of love that Panditji had for our children?

"What sort of a country are we that cannot protect our children from the machinations and manipulations of the most corrupt industry in the whole world? Yes Sir, the Global Corruption Report 2005 has stated

categorically that the $3100 billion medical industry is the most corrupt industry in the world. And yet we continue to pour billions down the throat of this monster. This corrupt industry is headed by the WHO, the UN, and the US based FDA and CDC whose shenanigans are now being probed by investigative journalists and the reports find place in such prestigious newspapers like the New York Times, The Guardian, and even The Lancet, one of the most prestigious medical journals of our times.

"The people all over the world are pointing out the flaws and fallacies of this industry. In the US it has been revealed that 783,936 people die every year due to medical malpractice, more than the combined number that die from road accidents and terrorist attacks. In India, the doctors say that in our towns alone 200,000 people die every year from adverse drug reactions, and 80,000 due to medical malpractices.

"In the TV channels we watch in horror as the doctors kill children in the womb, burn new born infants in the cots, cut the limbs of healthy people at the instance of the beggar mafia, trade in organs of the innocents, photograph female patients in the raw and sell the footage to the porn industry, and experiment new drugs and vaccines on eight-days old toddlers and infants in the creches. Recently all of India has been shocked at front-page headlines that said that the JE vaccine has already killed 22 children and seriously affected 504 others.

"How long will this go on, Sir? How long before this vile so-called science is replaced by more humane methods of treatment? Why should we be forced to be perennial guinea pigs at the hands of doctors who

openly admit that they are clueless as to why epidemics of chronic autoimmune disorders are spreading like wildfire across the world?

"It is said that in a society where people are unjustly imprisoned, the true place for a just man is also a prison. Therefore I request you, Sir, that we vaccine victims and other victims of the medical industry be arrested en masse and put behind bars. At least it will relieve us of the tension of seeing infants and adults being recklessly and systematically mauled in the hands of the cannibalistic medical industry.

"Please forgive me for being emotional. But after 27 years of personal suffering and the realization that things are not going to change despite our protests, I am finding it difficult to keep my mouth shut.

"President Sir, once again we appeal to you, please intervene and save our children. Please ensure that 1.74 million autistic children of India, who have been incapacitated by the use of mercury and aluminum in vaccines and the use of live measles virus, and of uncounted others who have died or rendered disabled due to toxic vaccine ingredients get the attention they deserve and that their parents are at least helped financially to ensure that their children are rehabilitated and lead some semblance of normal life after they are gone." (Note: Aluminum is 4000 times more toxic than lead!)

"Is this too much to ask of you, Sir?"

Respectfully yours,

Jagannath Chatterjee,

Vaccine damage victim,

Health Reform Activist.

(Vaccinations, Yahoo Groups)

Wednesday, 30 August 2006 (NWBC 202) Protests in India and

China against vaccinations

****

From the Idaho Observer November 15, 2005

8. To the Editor:

"My Uncle had been on a regimen of many medicines for several years. Heart pills, blood pressure pills, gout medicine and other drugs for prevention or control of various disorders. When he developed stomach cancer, the primary disease well documented by the Faulkner Hospital in Boston, MA, I attributed it to the many drugs he was using. Doctors adamantly disagreed and put him on chemotherapy which they discontinued after my uncle suffered a heart attack within hours after his second treatment. The chemotherapy was discontinued; but my uncle was told to continue with his usual drug therapy that consisted of 9 pills a day.

"At this time, without the Doctor's knowledge or consent, I convinced my uncle to embark on an alkaline diet. A diet consisting mainly of fruit and vegetables, and one that disallowed the use of any medicines. Within a

few weeks an endoscopy showed that the cancer was completely gone.

"Months have gone by. My uncle still goes in for checkups. The cancer is gone. He has never returned to the pills that the doctors insist he could not do without. To this day the doctors assume he is still on his prescribed medications. We hesitate to tell them the truth since we still believe that some forms of medical treatment are beneficial and we would not want to alienate the doctors or the insurance provider.

"Years have gone by. My uncle, now at age 89, welcomes any investigation into this matter, and is living proof that the pills he was taking, as many as 270 a month, were not only unnecessary, but harmful, since his vital signs are now better than ever.

"In my opinion, this is a cancer breakthrough. Herein may lay the answer to the health care crisis. Herein may lay the answer to why a rich nation is made to grovel. Herein lies the question, Has the Medical Industry grown so powerful and self-centered as to become a danger to our society?"

Bob Catalano

****

Vaccination Letter

"I am a moderator of an epilepsy group and I am so saddened at how many parents keep coming to our group due to seizures after vaccinations. I know personally what it is like to have a child with uncontrollable seizures all day long. It is so hard for me to understand why the big issue with vaccine dangers is always autism, but the other conditions are "swept

under the rug". I know autism affects a larger number of kids. When I have spoken with new parents about vaccinations, they are falsely assuming that since mercury has been taken out of vaccines, they do not have to worry about autism. But what about everything else? Is this the type of thing that people have to wait until it happens to them before they will take notice?"
Stephanie Precourt, Yahoo Vaccination Group

****
*

A message from Bernard Rimland, Ph.D.

"Parents: You can make a difference! You MUST make a difference! "Big Pharma has more paid lobbyists in Washington than there are Senators and Representatives. And they have lots of money and lots of influence. "But we have Right on our side, and sincerity, and dedication. We can't let Pharma win. The stakes are high We must win this battle, for our children and for ourselves.

"Make appointments to see your Senators and Representatives. Tell them: "We have no faith in the integrity of the CDC and the FDA. They are doing all they can to protect themselves and Big Pharma from the truth. That the autism epidemic is caused by Big Pharma's greed and the failure of the CDC and the FDA to do their jobs.

"Big Pharma must not be allowed to evade its financial liability for the damage their vaccines have caused. Like the tobacco companies in the last century, which kept denying the cigarette-lung cancer link, the drug companies are lying â€" with the help of the CDC and FDA â€" about the role of vaccines in causing the

autism's epidemic. When the lung cancer cases finally got to court, the truth came out. We parents insist on our right to hold the drug companies liable, in court, for the harm they have caused. The matter must be decided fairly in the legal system, and not by loophole riders exonerating the drug companies that have been added to appropriation bills in the dark of night. The drug companies caused the autism epidemic and they, not the parents nor the public, must pay the costs. They are guilty, they are very profitable and can and should be held accountable."

Very Sincerely,

Bernard Rimland, Ph.D., Director

Autism Research Institute

9. Index

AVI BioPharma, 51
AZT treatment, 51

Baxter, 51–52
Biblowit, Myra, 87
biopsies, 73, 82, 86
bird flu. *See* avian flu
  vaccine
birth defects, 39
Blackwell, Tom, 105
bloodstream, 3. *See also*
  immune system
Bolen, Tim, 35
Brackett, Cori, 59
breast cancer, 85–87
Breast Cancer Research
  Foundation, 87
Britain, vaccination
  programs in, 57
Burke, Fionnuala, 107–8
Burr, Richard, 67
Bush, George W., 45–47,
  49, 55, 60–62, 66–67

campaign contributions, by
  medical industry, 45, 63
Canada, vaccination
  programs in, 105, 110
cancer, 81–93
  case histories, 131–32
  immune system and,
    81–84, 87–88, 90
  non-medical treatment
    of, 21–22
  rates of, 88
  research, profit motive
    and, 84–87
  role of drugs in, 83,
    88–89

treatments for, 6–8, 10
  tumor injury role, 73, 82,
    86
Cancer Research Institute,
  86
Cantwell, Alan, Jr., 88–89
Carmen Balber, Jamie
  Court, 52–53, 67
Center fro Public Integrity,
  5–6
Centers for Disease Control
  and Prevention (CDC), 18,
  36–37, 110, 133
Cerebral Palsy, 39
cervical cancer vaccine,
  36–37, 75–77
Chan, Margaret, 50
Chatterjee, Jagannath,
  123–27
chemotherapy treatment,
  7–8, 83, 131–32
Child Protective Services,
  40
children's issues, 21, 37–
  40. *See also* vaccinations
China, vaccination
  programs in, 104–5
Chipman, James, 107
Christian Scientists, 109
Clinton, Hilary, 66
complications, as cause of
  death, 16
Congress. *See* United
  States government
consumerism, 3–4, 17,
  34–35
corruption, 90–93, 124–25
crib death, 101, 113–15
Cummings, Bill, 64–66